'YOU MADE THE DECISION.
HERE ARE SOME MORE "POWER" TOOLS.'

Dr Phil sent you a major, scientifically based
wake-up call. Now, here are even more daily tools for
living the ultimate choice to take control of your weight –
instead of letting your weight control you. You can do it –
and Dr Phil has some important nutritional plans to
make it even more manageable.

In this essential companion to *The Ultimate Weight Solution*,
Dr Phil takes his groundbreaking weight loss plan
even further by giving you a wealth of handy, accessible
advice for every food situation and decision that you face.
Here are the hands-on tools to help you identify
WHAT TO EAT
WHEN TO EAT
WHERE TO EAT
HOW TO EAT
WHY TO EAT OR NOT EAT

and essential, straightforward information on
THE CALORIE COUNTS FOR HIGH- AND
LOW-RESPONSE COST FOODS

UNHEALTHY HUNGER-DRIVING FOODS TO AVOID
WHILE IN THE WEIGHT LOSS MODE

AT-A-GLANCE FOOD COMPARISONS

HIGH-RESPONSE COST, HUNGER-SUPPRESSING FOODS

TAKE-AWAY & RESTAURANT FOOD STRATEGIES
and much more!

ALSO BY DR PHIL MCGRAW

Life Strategies
Life Strategies Workbook
Relationship Rescue
Relationship Rescue Workbook
Self Matters
The Self Matters Companion
The Ultimate Weight Solution
The Ultimate Weight Solution Cookbook
Family First

The Ultimate
Weight Solution
Food Guide

Dr Phil McGraw

POCKET BOOKS
New York   London   Toronto   Sydney

First published in Great Britain by Pocket Books, 2005
An imprint of Simon & Schuster UK Ltd
A Viacom Company

1   3   5   7   9   10   8   6   4   2

Simon & Schuster UK Ltd
Africa House
64–78 Kingsway
London WC2B 6AH

www.simonsays.co.uk

Simon & Schuster Australia
Sydney

A CIP catalogue record for this book is available from the British Library

ISBN 1-4165-0208-4
EAN 9781416502081

Printed and bound in Great Britain by Cox & Wyman

This book is dedicated to the millions of people who are using The Ultimate Weight Solution *and changing the epidemic of obesity, one life at a time.*

Acknowledgements

One of the best decisions I have ever made was to ask Maggie Robinson, Ph.D., to be a part of my crusade of tackling obesity in America. Maggie is clearly the pre-eminent nutritionist in America today, and her tireless work on content, organization, flow, and writing was an invaluable asset to this project. Thanks, Maggie, for lending your expertise and passion about nutritional science to *The Ultimate Weight Solution Food Guide*. You have taught me a tremendous amount and I am proud to call you a friend.

Acknowledgements

Contents

The Ultimate
Weight Solution
Food Guide

Introduction

Get excited.

What you are holding in your hands is a powerful tool for change, one that will help you take your nutrition, and your eating, to an entirely new level of self-control. If you take what I have to say about nutrition and food in this guide, learn it, and put it to use, you can keep your momentum going in the direction of permanent weight loss. I know that is the result you're aiming for, so let's plan to further that momentum of success right now.

If you have read or are reading *The Ultimate Weight Solution: The 7 Keys to Weight Loss Freedom*, then you have taken a very important step towards success. You know that losing weight and keeping it off are not simply matters of eating less and exercising more (although both are crucial), but of changing the particular psychological, behavioural, and environmental factors that cause you to overeat in the first place. You know you must build a way of life that supports healthy weight management on every side. Everything you will find in *The Ultimate Weight Solution*, and in this companion guide, is based on the premise that the power to change your weight and your health lies solely within you.

And if you are among the millions of people who are using the seven keys to weight loss freedom, then I am happy for you and proud of what you are doing to maximize your life. You are on the path to living a life that is infinitely more healthy for you, with an outpouring of positives because you have had the courage to do something significant and rewarding for yourself.

When you use the seven keys, you begin to: rid yourself of wrong thinking, heal yourself of emotions standing in the way of a healthy relationship with food, create a no-fail environment, shape your eating behaviour into what you need for lifetime weight control, get real about nutritional choices that worked to your detriment, change your priorities to include exercise, and plug into a circle of support for encouragement and accountability. In short, you are changing how you're living.

Part of this process involves getting real about all those fad, 'flavour-of-the-month' type diets you tried in the past – diets that promised you a shortcut but sent you down a dead-end road to failure instead. These diets can leave you weighing in much heavier than usual, with a pile-up of not just pounds, but discouragement over your repeated failures. The promises made by fad diets can be seductive, and I assure you that caving in to them is a short drop back into the frustration and weight from where you came.

The current preoccupation with ultra low-carbohydrate dieting is of deep concern to me as a clinical and medical psychologist. What is so troubling from both a psychological and nutritional perspective is that most of these diets advocate eating less than 100 grams of carbohydrates a day, when in fact your body requires nearly double that amount for normal brain metabolism and muscle function.

When you deny your body and brain sufficient carbohydrates, it can damage your inner psychology. It can bring on fatigue, irritability, and mood changes. Why? Under normal circumstances, your brain uses roughly 500 calories' worth of carbohydrate a day for optimal functioning, including the production of brain chemicals responsible for feelings of mental well-being. So without carbohydrates, your mental and emotional edge is gravely affected. Think of the consequences if you are an emotional overeater who decides to follow a low-carbohydrate diet. You already have a habit of medicating yourself with food. Then comes the double whammy: you choose to diet in such a way that it makes you feel worse emotionally and now you are more vulnerable than ever to bingeing and overeating. You are, in essence, conspiring against yourself by choosing a diet that without question sets you up for failure by further weakening you where you are the weakest. You are creating obstacles for yourself that you don't need.

It is time for all this health-defeating, behaviour-defeating pseudonutrition to stop. Nutritionally, the solution for successful weight loss is not ultra low-carbohydrate dieting – far from it. What can genuinely help you lose weight and keep it off is *moderate* nutrition across the board – moderate carbohydrates, moderate protein, and moderate fat, and this current, accurate information comes straight from nutritional scientists, not from weight loss gurus or food faddists.

So with *The Ultimate Weight Solution Food Guide*, I am back with more to say about diet and nutrition – what to eat, how to eat, and why, in order to help you do what no fad diet has ever accomplished, and that is achieve lifelong weight control. In this guide, you won't be relying on bad nutritional information, but rather on sound techniques and principles for shedding weight permanently by taking a moderate, balanced approach to eating.

In the first part of this guide, I have set out for you an effective, highly structured three-stage food plan, including weeks and weeks of menus, that takes you from initial weight loss right through to maintenance. It includes:

- **My Rapid Start Plan,** a specialized 14-day approach to eating that activates early, immediate weight loss in order to reinforce, and create for you, a pattern of success that sets the stage for continued weight loss. In this stage, you'll be eating foods in their pure, mostly unprocessed state (raw fruits, raw vegetables, vegetables cooked from raw or from frozen, and certain wholegrains). This helps clear your system of processed sugars and refined carbohydrates in order to restore better metabolic control and recondition your taste preferences for healthier, more wholesome foods. Your body will begin changing for the better in a matter of days.

- **My High-Response Cost, High-Yield Weight Loss Plan,** for sustainable, consistent weight loss without deprivation. This stage liberalizes your eating plan, while remaining effectively calorie-controlled to ensure steady weight loss. There are no holes in your nutrition either, only moderate, balanced eating with foods that offer built-in protection from gaining weight, some of which you can eat to your heart's content.

- **My Ultimate Maintenance Plan,** in which we will work through a number of critical steps so that you can learn how to live in your new body. With this plan, you'll be able to stay at your newfound thin, fit self for a lifetime as long as you do what is required.

The second part of *The Ultimate Weight Solution Food Guide* is devoted to a comprehensive listing of the nutrient content of thousands of foods, divided into my classifications of high-response cost, high-yield foods and low-response cost, low-yield foods. For you to make healthier nutritional choices, you need to know what's in the foods you're choosing, from calories to carbohydrates, from fat to sodium. This part of the guide provides that information, in one easy-to-use reference.

This guide is designed to be used along with *The Ultimate Weight Solution*, which provides the keys and their corresponding steps to help you create a new lifestyle for yourself that is consistent with whatever it takes to support long-term rather than quick-fix weight loss. The guide helps you keep your nutritional momentum going, building on and adding to the book, with action-oriented answers and clear-cut instructions on exactly what and how to eat.

Throughout this guide, you will be introduced to even more behavioural and nutritional strategies, in order to support you when you're not in the mood to stick to your plan. Successful weight management isn't about will-power. It's about creating a life programme by controlling, among other things, your environment, your schedule, and your self-destructive behaviours. The more strategies you can plug into your life, the more successful you will be.

You know from personal experience that there is nothing more frustrating, or more disheartening, than the struggle to lose weight and keep it off. Probably more than anything right now, you want to put that part of you behind you – and start piecing your life back together in such a way that you can respect and like yourself for who you are and what you do. And if you haven't said so to yourself, let me say it for you: you deserve more out of life than the way you have been living.

I am here to tell you that this want is worth having, and that you are worth whatever it takes to get it. This guide is thus a worthy resource for a worthy cause – you! The information on every page will help you, if you choose to help yourself to what it has to offer. It will not make you lose pounds or trim inches. Only you can do that. You have within you everything you need to transform the life you've been living, and become the healthy *you* that you want to be. Now is your chance to make a better life for yourself. It's a chance you don't want to miss!

ONE

Putting Your Weight on Project Status

You have made the important decision to lose weight, and you want to do it right this time. But to do so, you must be willing to put your weight on what I like to call Project Status. This means that you must consciously decide to work actively and purposely on improving your weight and your fitness level each and every day. Putting your weight on Project Status means giving your health and vitality a new, higher priority in your life, such that they become of conscious importance to you. You stay committed to working on them, disciplining yourself by working on all seven keys to weight loss freedom. (I've summarized the keys for you in the box on pages 25–26.)

You get out of this project – your weight – what you put into it. It will be from your commitment to set a personal standard for yourself – one that says you will not quit and you will not push aside your goals for a trimmer, healthier body – that your success will follow. You must be willing to reach for what you want and reach right now. To be in Project Status means that you do not neglect to take care of yourself first, and now is the time to start doing that.

Before beginning the nutritional plan in this guide, you must take some essential first steps that will help you reach the peak of your effectiveness, and lay the groundwork for constructive, lasting change. This is very important – don't hurry through these initial steps or avoid this part of the process. Take it seriously, and I promise you that you will have the foundation for the most effective and dramatic changes you have ever made in your weight.

Step 1:
Determine your Get-Real Weight.

Your get-real weight is the healthiest and most realistic weight for you, based on your height, your bone structure, and your sex. It is not necessarily the weight of your youth, but rather a state of health and well-being that is congruent and in harmony with how you are physically and genetically configured. It is the weight that is 'right' for you – a stable, comfortable weight, at which you look good, feel good, and lovingly accept yourself from the inside out.

You can figure out your get-real weight by using my Body Weight Standards, a system I developed for my patients; it is a modified and more realistic version of height–weight tables. Though not perfect, these body weight standards are more reflective of what can be achieved and certainly a better measure of where most people should be, weight-wise.

Using the Body Weight Standards chart below, identify where you should be, so that you can move forward from where you are now. The lower end of the ranges are for small-boned

DR PHIL'S BODY WEIGHT STANDARDS

Height	Women	Men
4' 10"	90 – **100** – 110	114 – **127** – 140
4' 11"	95 – **105** – 116	119 – **132** – 145
5'	99 – **110** – 121	123 – **137** – 151
5' 1"	103 – **115** – 127	128 – **142** – 156
5' 2"	108 – **120** – 132	132 – **147** – 162
5' 3"	112 – **125** – 138	137 – **152** – 167
5' 4"	117 – **130** – 143	141 – **157** – 173
5' 5"	122 – **135** – 148	146 – **162** – 178
5' 6"	126 – **140** – 154	150 – **167** – 184
5' 7"	130 – **145** – 160	155 – **172** – 189
5' 8"	135 – **150** – 165	159 – **177** – 195
5' 9"	139 – **155** – 171	164 – **182** – 200
5' 10"	144 – **160** – 176	168 – **187** – 206
5' 11"	148 – **165** – 182	173 – **192** – 211
6'	153 – **170** – 187	177 – **197** – 217
6' 1"	157 – **175** – 193	182 – **202** – 222
6' 2"	162 – **180** – 198	186 – **207** – 228
6' 3"	166 – **185** – 204	191 – **212** – 233
6' 4"	171 – **190** – 209	195 – **217** – 239

My get-real weight is: _____

people; the upper end, for larger-boned individuals. Be honest here: don't subjectively say you are small-boned when, in fact, you are just the opposite. Your get-real weight is your target. Record it in the space above.

STEP 2:
CHECK AND RECORD YOUR CURRENT WEIGHT AND WAIST MEASUREMENT BEFORE YOU START.

Do two things: first, step on the scales to weigh yourself to determine your starting point. Then, measure your waist with a tape measure positioned 2.5 cm/1 inch above your navel. Taking waist measurements is important because weight distribution – where you carry weight on your body – can affect your health, for better or for worse. A too-large waistline circumference, for example, places you at greater risk for heart disease, diabetes, and certain cancers.

A waist measurement of 89 cm/35 inches or more for women and 102 cm/40 inches or more for men is cause for concern and may indicate that you are at risk for heart disease or diabetes. Keeping tabs on this simple measurement can protect you in some important ways.

Write your weight and waist measurement in the space below, along with the date.

Date: _____
My weight: _____
My waist measurement: _____

Although I do not advocate obsessive weighing and measuring, you do need to monitor your progress towards your get-real weight with some regularity and reasonable frequency. You should weigh yourself at least at one- or two-week intervals to stay on target; then record your weight in a notebook or journal. The scales should show a weight loss that may be quite dramatic in the beginning, eventually tapering off to a steady, even loss of a few pounds each week. If you aren't dropping pounds at a steady rate, or if you gain weight, you should be motivated to course-correct some aspect of the weight loss plan to make it more effective, including changing your behaviour so that it is harder for you to cheat.

Weigh yourself at the same time each week, because your weight fluctuates throughout the day, and you can weigh more at night than you do in the morning. Promise yourself you will not self-destruct if the scales move up a few pounds, but instead make this a priority for action-oriented repair.

At monthly intervals, remeasure your waist and record these measurements. Watching your pounds and inches diminish will help reinforce your resolve and keep you moving in the right direction.

STEP 3:
CLEAR YOUR ENVIRONMENT OF 'LOW-RESPONSE COST, LOW-YIELD FOODS'.

The presence of food is one of the most insistent of all triggers to eat or overeat, and you know this yourself if you have ever tried to sample just a few healthy items from a buffet table. This step is thus about removing tempting foods from your environment, including your home, office, car, or anywhere you store food. After all, you can't eat what is not there.

Specifically, I would like you to take an inventory of your environment, looking for and tossing out what I call 'low-response cost, low-yield foods'. So that you understand the terminology, these foods require very little *response* from you when you eat them. In plain terms, they are foods that you just gulp and gain – easily ingested, overly convenient, and requiring little or no preparation on your part.

An excellent example of a low-response cost food is a microwaveable sandwich. You zap it in your microwave in a matter of seconds, no preparation required. When you eat it, you don't even have to chomp on it; it just slithers down your throat in a few quick gulps. What happens is that you consume an incredibly high number of calories and fat in a very short period of time.

Most low-response cost foods are also *low-yield foods*. That means they provide very little in the way of good nutrition, with a lot of calories packed into a very small amount of food. Sugar is an example of a low-yield food. It is very high in calories but practically devoid of nutrition, and for these reasons, it is best kept off-limits if you want to control your weight successfully.

Low-yield foods are engineered to be addictive; loaded with sugar, extra fat, calories, too much salt, and unhealthy additives; and of questionable nutritional value. What's more, they are processed and refined; that is, they have been milled or altered in some fashion that devalues their nutrition by extracting fibre and other nutrients.

To sum up, low-response cost, low-yield foods:
- Invite and promote fast, uncontrollable eating.
- Need little or no preparation time.
- Require little chewing or effort to eat. The food slides down your throat, and you barely have to chew it.
- Melt in your mouth.
- Can be too easily eaten straight from a package or container.
- Are highly processed.
- Are light on nutrition.

One of the most offending characteristics of low-response cost, low-yield foods is that they are *hunger drivers*. These foods do not keep you satisfied for very long and may make you hungrier later. Here's why: after you eat these foods, your body's natural stop-eating signals don't even have time to kick in. It takes about twenty minutes from the time you eat something until the hypothalamus in your brain shuts off your appetite. There's absolutely no way that microwaved sandwich can offer any satisfying effects when it's overly easy to wolf it down in a matter of seconds. So you keep eating more and more of this stuff until you've eaten way beyond the point of fullness; and the unfortunate fact is that you're overfed with unnecessary calories and fat.

On pages 358 to 545 of this food guide, you'll find a comprehensive listing of low-response cost, low-yield foods by category. These are foods you want to limit or avoid. For now, here is an abbreviated list that will give you an idea of what to toss out:

- Biscuits, sweets, and any high-calorie, sweetened snack foods.
- Salty foods such as crisps, pretzels, tortilla chips, nuts, and other packaged snacks.
- Pastries and doughnuts.
- Cakes, snack cakes, pies, and other baked goods.
- Pre-sweetened, sugary breakfast cereals.
- White bread, white rolls, white baps – anything that is not wholegrain.
- Biscuits that are not wholegrain.
- Processed sliced meats.
- Ice cream and high-sugar frozen desserts.
- Quick-fix prepared foods such as pizza, fried main courses and dinners, and microwaveable sandwiches.
- Syrups, jams, and jellies.

- High-fat spreads, peanut butter, and dips.
- Sugared fizzy drinks and beverages, including flavoured coffees.
- Alcoholic beverages.
- Any packaged food in which sugar is listed as one of the first three ingredients.
- Any food that can be classified as 'junk food'.
- Any food that you habitually binge on.

Ridding your environment of low-response cost, low-yield foods is one of the best moves you can take towards setting yourself up for success. It helps you get past needing to feel motivated all the time to try to lose weight. When your enthusiasm flags and your will-power conks out – which it will – you need to have your environment set up in such a way that it supports you. This crucial step of eliminating low-response cost, low-yield foods does this for you.

STEP 4.
STOCK YOUR KITCHEN WITH 'HIGH-RESPONSE COST, HIGH-YIELD FOODS'.

By 'high-response cost foods', I mean foods that require a great deal of work and effort to prepare and to eat. The work output, or *response* on your part, that is required to ingest these foods is high, whereas the calorie payoff – although healthy – is low. A good example of a high-response cost, high-yield food is a ripe, juicy apple. It is coarse and takes a lot of chewing and grinding to get it down. It is also packed with fibre, which keeps your stomach from emptying too rapidly.

Why is this important? The fact that you must take time to

prepare these foods, and that they take effort to chew, eat, and digest, is a real advantage to weight control. Why? *Because high-response cost foods defeat the urge to eat on impulse and therefore support better control.*

High-response cost foods are thus *hunger suppressors*, meaning they can control and curb your hunger. Because they take longer to eat, your body has more time to receive stop-eating signals from your hypothalamus. By the time you chew and ingest these foods, you're starting to feel full, so there is little chance that you will overeat. You will be amazed at how little food you'll eat, yet how full and satisfied you'll feel after eating it.

Most high-response cost foods also happen to be 'high-yield foods'. High-yield foods are those that supply a lot of nutrients – in the form of carbohydrates, protein, fat, vitamins, minerals, fibre, and other food components – relative to the low amount of calories they contain.

High-yield foods are generally those of a more pure, basic variety and are closer to the state in which they are found in nature. They have not been critically changed during food processing, and thus are not usually laced with added sugar, fat, additives, and other health-defeating ingredients. High-yield foods are abundant in fibre, a weight-control ally that promotes feelings of fullness, stabilizes your blood sugar, and thus keeps your hunger at bay so that you're less likely to overeat.

High-yield foods such as fruits and vegetables are colourful too, a sign that they are plentiful in important food factors that reduce your risk of disease.

To recap, high-response cost, high-yield foods are those that:

- Take time and effort to prepare.
- Require a great deal of chewing and ingestion energy.
- Cannot be eaten quickly.

- Suppress your hunger and curb your cravings.
- Are not 'convenience foods' in any sense of the word.
- Supply a healthy balance of vitamins, minerals, fibre, and other nutrients.

For successful weight control, stock your kitchen with high-response cost, high-yield foods. There is a comprehensive list of these foods starting on page 150, and you should become very familiar with them because they form the centrepiece of nutrition for healthy weight control. For now, and as you begin this plan, make sure you have these foods on hand:

- Poultry, such as chicken and turkey breasts (prepared without skin).
- Fresh, frozen, or canned seafood (nothing that is breaded, however).
- Lean cuts of meat.
- Fresh eggs.
- Fresh fruits and vegetables. Frozen is fine too, since they've been chilled immediately after harvesting and may contain more nutrients than fresh produce that has been sitting on the shelf or in your refrigerator. Canned fruits and vegetables are acceptable, but may contain high levels of sodium.
- Wholegrains and cereals, such as brown rice, bulgur wheat, oatmeal, rice, barley, and millet.
- High-fibre cereals. Although a packaged product, these cereals are specially formulated with added fibre – a hunger-suppressing ingredient in high-response cost grains and cereals.
- Reduced fat or fat-free dairy products such as skimmed milk, semi-skimmed milk, sugar-free yogurt, and low-fat cheeses.

- Healthy fats such as olive oil, rapeseed oil, and nuts and seeds. These fats appear to delay hunger and help you feel more satisfied after eating a meal that contains them.

(For a comparative look at hunger suppressors and hunger drivers, refer to the chart on page 24.)

STEP 5:
PRIORITIZE EXERCISE IN YOUR LIFE.

The fit, in-shape people of this world are doing something right – that something is exercise. Exercise burns calories; in fact, you can lose a pound of fat in ten exercise sessions of approximately forty-five minutes to one hour each, provided you do not take in a surplus of calories. The more food you burn off through exercise, the less you store as fat. Exercise also accelerates your metabolism, the physiological process that converts food into energy, so that you are burning up more calories even at rest.

There's something else at work, too: food behaviour and exercise behaviour are highly interactive, with a powerful connection operating between the two. If you exercise on a regular basis, a rather amazing phenomenon occurs: you'll begin to experience a weakening desire to overeat. Your food behaviour will begin to change almost automatically, and you'll make healthier food choices as a matter of routine.

For effective weight control, it is best to start an established exercise programme that involves three to four hours a week of aerobic activity such as brisk walking, biking, jogging, aerobic dancing, playing tennis, aerobic exercise machines (treadmill, stair-climber, and so forth), or swimming.

Added to your aerobic exercise programme should be weight training, at least two to three times a week. Weight training just happens to be one of the most powerful ways to rejuvenate and speed up your metabolism. It helps burn body fat (nearly 100 per cent of the weight you lose is pure fat if you weight-train). And it builds firm, well-developed muscle while you're losing weight. More muscle translates into a faster metabolism. The reason for this is that muscle tissue demands much more oxygen and calories to sustain itself than fat tissue does. Fat tissue, by contrast, is relatively inactive, while muscle is constantly burning fuel at a rapid rate even while you're at rest. When you add muscle to your body through weight training, your metabolic rate goes up and stays up twenty-four hours a day.

Weight training also makes maintaining your weight loss much easier and more automatic. In fact, a number of studies have found that weight training stands out as a proven lifestyle strategy for keeping excess weight off over the long term. So for healthy, ongoing weight management, you need to consider weight training.

Supporting your weight loss by exercising is a real chance for you to get permanent control of your weight, no matter how long it has been since you last exercised.

STEP 6:
CREATE ACCOUNTABILITY.

The next important step before getting started requires that you make yourself accountable with regard to your get-real goal weight. This means enlisting someone who will serve as your 'teammate', someone to whom you commit to make periodic reports. This person should come from your relational circle of support (explained in key 7): family members and friends whom you consider to be the closest people in your life – the people you trust and value most. Figure out who would most strongly support what you want to accomplish and who would be willing and available to act in this capacity. Your teammate will be the person to whom you will have to confess if you fail to do what you plan to do.

At least once a week, if not daily, report on your compliance with your food plan, your exercise progress, the number of pounds you've lost, or other measures of progress. Knowing that you will check in with someone tomorrow keeps you on track today.

YOUR PERSONALIZED FOOD DIARY

When you start this plan, keep a 'personalized food diary' in which you accurately record everything you eat and drink, as well as other elements of relevance, such as your energy intake (calories). Whether you like it or not, calories still do count when it comes to weight control, so you do need to pay some degree of attention to how many calories you're taking in. Now don't lock up on me here. I am not asking you to become tediously preoccupied with counting calories. What I am suggesting is that you keep track of your calories for perhaps just a week or two, in order to make sure that you are not overindulging on overlooked calories.

Becoming knowledgeable about the calorie counts of foods you typically eat helps keep you on track in terms of how much you're eating. The calorie information in this food guide will provide valuable, at-your-fingertips reference material for doing that.

Use the Food Diary to Plan Your Meals

One important way to use the personalized food diary below is to pre-plan what you will eat and drink each day. By this, I mean that you commit to paper your menu for the day, including three meals and two snacks, then eat only the foods on that menu. The significance of having a food plan, prepared ahead of time, is that it frees you from making last-minute decisions about what to eat and prevents you from caving in to sudden impulses to overeat. Planning your eating in advance eliminates any doubt about what you will eat and removes your fear of losing control. With a food plan in place for the day, you can and will regain greater control over your eating. So use this diary as a meal planner, above all.

Use the Food Diary to Monitor Your Eating Behaviour

But you do not have to stop there. You can use this diary to record important information about your nutrition and eating habits. For example, you can record the time of your meals, the place, what you were doing at the time, or, in some cases, the emotional states (happy, sad, lonely, bored, stressed, angry, etc.) that may have triggered you to eat 'off plan'.

This information can help you see, in unquestionable black and white, precisely which eating habits you need to adjust or high-risk situations that are sabotaging your efforts. Maybe you find that you mindlessly reach for foods such as biscuits, cake, sweets, or ice cream – the so-called 'comfort foods' – when you feel tired after a long day at work. Or that being in certain places, like your car or office, triggers the impulse to eat.

Then you can thoughtfully review your entries, looking for

red flags. Assess the obstacles that can have an impact on reaching your get-real weight. This means anticipating the times, places, circumstances – even people – that typically make it difficult for you to stay the course. That way, you can work out an advance strategy for avoiding these pitfalls, or at least outlasting them. You're in a better position to avoid them by changing your routine, changing your schedule, or changing your environment.

You can also plan very carefully what you are going to do at those moments when you have the urge to binge or overeat. This should involve 'incompatible substitutes' – activities such as exercising, relaxation, listening to music – any activity that cannot coexist with eating. For example, when you feel compelled to soothe frustrations with a bag of crisps, pick up your knitting needles instead and start knitting. Knitting is incompatible with crunching down on crisps. Or take a walk. Walking around the block is incompatible with bingeing. Incompatible substitutes also take your mind off food and eating. So as soon as you feel the impulse, begin engaging, deliberately, in the incompatible substitute.

Keeping this food diary is crucial to the process of losing weight. It is a vital part of what psychologists call 'self-monitoring', a way to keep tabs on your progress and performance – not only to see where you need to take corrective action, but also to highlight the positive changes you're making. People who self-monitor their behaviour are more successful at losing weight and keeping it off than those who choose not to self-monitor. So let me encourage you to self-monitor. What you do not acknowledge is only going to get worse until you do.

On the following page is a sample diary. You should make as many photocopies as you need of this page. You don't have to use the diary forever – just long enough for you to see what's

Personalized Food Diary

Day of Week: _____

Date: _____

Time	Food Eaten	Amount	Compliance	Calories	Place	Circumstances

working and what's not – and to get the hang of what you need to be correcting on a day-to-day basis so that you can take important and timely coping steps.

Remember, you can use this diary as a meal planner to map out your meals for the next day, and as a log to identify correctable aspects of your behaviour that you need to change. To help you fill this out, here are some important instructions:

- In column 1 *(time)*, record the time of day you plan to eat. If you do not know when you'll be eating, write down 'breakfast', 'lunch', 'dinner' and 'snacks'.

- In column 2 *(food eaten)*, describe your meal or snack. Write down everything you plan to eat at those meals. If you eat something you have not planned to eat, write that down as soon as possible afterwards. (Note the time in the first column, too.) Leave nothing out.

- In column 3 *(amount)*, write down how much you ate (the amount or portion size).

- In column 4 *(compliance)*, note whether your meal or snack complied with your planned menu. Place a check mark in the allotted space if it did.

- In column 5 *(calories)*, write down the calories you consumed for each meal or snack. Add up your calories at the end of each day. (Remember, you do not have to do this forever – just long enough to get a feel for how well you're doing. Just a few days of calculating your calories can pinpoint overlooked sources of calories, plus provide some excellent nutritional self-diagnosis.)

- In column 6 *(place)*, note where you were at the time of the meal or snack – at your dining-room table, in the kitchen, watching television, in your car, at your desk, at a social occasion, or at a restaurant, for example.

- In column 7 (*circumstances*), describe any noteworthy circumstances surrounding the meal or snack, such as your feelings or emotions, whether you felt tired or unusually hungry, or if the meal happened in response to a stressful event.

If you have taken the above steps to put your weight on project status, you are ready to move on. Using the nutritional strategies that follow, you will be able to reprogram yourself for success rather than failure. Rewards will start rolling in quicker than you think. Your weight control experience will no longer be characterized by wasted moments and frustration, but by a sense of triumph and mastery. It's time to go for it.

Hunger Suppressors

- Lean animal-based proteins such as fish, meat, and poultry
- Fresh fruits
- Fresh vegetables
- Beans and pulses (e.g., kidney beans, pinto beans, or black beans)
- Wholegrains and high-fibre cereals
- Soups, broth-based
- Healthy fats (such as olive oil, rapeseed oil, or flaxseed oil)
- Nuts and seeds, unsalted and preferably still in their hulls

Hunger Drivers

- Most fast foods
- Fizzy drinks and all sweetened beverages
- Alcoholic beverages
- Sugared cereals
- Ice cream and frozen desserts
- Sweets
- Salty foods such as snack foods (crisps, pretzels, salted nuts, snack mixes, etc.)
- Baked goods, including cakes, pastries, and doughnuts
- Any food classified as 'junk food'

THE 7 KEYS TO WEIGHT LOSS FREEDOM

Key 1 – Right Thinking. Lay aside self-defeating, invalid mind-sets that do not work. They have the power to keep you from making different choices or developing new behaviours. Too often, we let these negative notions go unchallenged, and we act as though they were true. You must monitor what you're thinking and challenge whether it is true. If it's not working, replace it with thinking that works.

Key 2 – Healing Feelings. Overcome emotional overeating by managing inappropriate reactions to stress; solving problems rather than dwelling on them; changing self-defeating thoughts, since more often than not, feelings follow thoughts; gaining closure on unfinished emotional business; and learning new ways to cope without resorting to food.

Key 3 – A No-Fail Environment. Design your world so that you can't help but succeed. This involves removing temptations to eat and rearranging your schedule in order to avoid or minimize triggers to overeat.

Key 4 – Mastery over Food and Impulse Eating. There's only one reason why you haven't changed the bad stuff in your life. You're getting something out of it. I'm not saying that you're getting something healthy or positive, but people do not continue in situations, attitudes, or actions that do not give them a payoff. This key helps you identify those payoffs, unplug from them, and replace bad habits with healthy behaviour.

Key 5 – High-Response Cost, High-Yield Nutrition. To lose weight, you must choose foods that support good behavioural control over your eating; that is, high-response cost, high-yield foods, organized into a moderate, balanced, calorie-controlled plan to ensure weight loss.

Key 6 – Intentional Exercise. Prioritize regular exercise into your life most days of the week – walking, jogging, aerobic dance classes, yoga, playing a sport, or lifting weights. Exercise does more than simply burn calories; it changes your self-perception so you stop labelling yourself as a couch potato.

Key 7 – Your Circle of Support. Surround yourself with supportive, like-minded people who want you to lose weight and succeed at your health and fitness efforts.

T W O

High-Response Cost, High-Yield Nutrition

A THREE-STAGE PLAN TO WEIGHT LOSS FREEDOM

Nutritionally, you need something doable but not drastic that you can do, starting today, to start dropping pounds and inches. This is exactly what this chapter is intended to help you do. What you are about to learn here is a workable, effective three-stage plan for taking weight off and keeping it off – a plan that is built around high-response cost, high-yield foods.

Why are these foods emphasized?

The answer to that is easy: from the perspective of weight management, high-response cost, high-yield foods support behavioural change. They encourage slow eating, they are tremendously satisfying, and they curb cravings and hunger pangs. Because high-response cost foods have not been critically changed during food processing, you do not have to worry about eating added sugar or fat – and suffering the weight-gaining side effects that those additions bring. In short, high-response cost, high-yield foods form the basis of a healthy, nutritious diet because they energize, protect, and build your body.

By contrast, low-response, low-yield foods lead to a considerable amount of mindless, uncontrollable overeating. If you eliminate or cut back on these foods, weight management becomes so much easier and requires far less vigilance over what and how you eat.

This three-stage plan provides total nutrition using everyday foods that are eaten in the real world, allowing you to live normally and at peace with food. It's easy to incorporate into your life, without turning it upside down or driving you nuts. It re-establishes normal patterns of eating behaviour so that you don't have to exercise such grit-your-teeth restraint, which is so often the undoing of dieters. This plan is something you can stick to for good, and its effect on your health can be transformative.

Learning, and putting into action, the three stages of my high-response cost, high-yield nutrition plan is at the absolute core of what you must do nutritionally for permanent weight loss. Here is how it works:

STAGE 1:
THE RAPID START PLAN

The Rapid Start Plan is a 14-day, calorie-controlled, carbohydrate-modified plan that helps gear your body for accelerated weight loss. It also initiates the process of *choice shift*, in which your taste preferences for high-sugar, high-fat foods begin to change to a preference for healthier foods. As you replace low-response cost, low-yield foods with healthier alternatives, for example, biscuits with apples, oranges, or some other healthy food, your preference for the healthier food becomes stronger and more appetizing. In unison with choice shift, you will also experience diminished cravings for sugar and refined carbohydrates.

When you change your diet with the goal of losing weight, the first initial weeks are absolutely critical. I know through personal experience from working with thousands of people who have been overweight or obese, in addition to valid nutritional research, that losing a significant amount of weight at the very outset of a programme can lay constructive groundwork for long-term success. In other words, *initial* weight loss has the chance to lead to *long-term* weight maintenance. If you get a running start on losing weight right away, expect to make it to the finish line as a winner.

The Rapid Start Plan has its genesis in my training as a medical psychologist working with the medical population of patients who were dealing with all of the problems and diseases secondary to obesity. The dietary strategies I designed for these patients enjoyed amazing results, and as a result, I got called on more and more to work with people who were overweight or obese – and so the basics of this nutritional plan were born.

The Rapid Start Plan gives you the freedom to eat a wide variety of food groups: lean proteins, fruits and dairy products (left out of most reducing diets), enough natural starches for energy, unlimited amounts of non-starchy vegetables, and a variety of healthy fats.

During your 14 days on the Rapid Start Plan:

1. Eat three regular meals a day (breakfast, lunch, and dinner) and two snacks. Try to schedule your meals at fairly regular times, whenever possible. This keeps your blood sugar steady, so that you're less vulnerable to

cravings. In addition, it helps you settle into a more disciplined eating pattern.

2. Have a protein serving at each of your three main meals. This breaks down to an egg, two egg whites, or 2 ounces of a lean turkey product (such as turkey bacon) for breakfast; 4 ounces of protein for lunch; and 4 ounces for dinner. Protein is a hunger suppressor and has a positive effect on metabolic activity.

3. Eat unlimited amounts (but at least four servings) of non-starchy vegetables (salad vegetables, broccoli, cauliflower, green beans, spinach, etc.) daily. These vegetables may be raw, or cooked from fresh or frozen. Eat these foods until you feel satisfied but not too full. Learn to tune in to your own hunger and fullness cues.

4. Modify your intake of starchy carbohydrates (potatoes, rice, wholegrains, high-fibre cereal, pulses, etc.) to one serving a day (for women) or two servings a day (for men, since men usually require more calories a day than women do). You'll be temporarily limiting these starchy foods (but not cutting them out altogether). Do not eat starchy carbohydrates after your midday meal. Most of your starchy carbohydrates in this stage are natural, unrefined choices – nothing remotely processed (such as bread or pasta).

5. Eat two servings of fresh fruit daily – but no fruit juice in this stage, because juice does little to help suppress your appetite.

6. Eat two servings of low-fat dairy foods daily. Often limited or cut out altogether in many diets, these foods furnish the bone-building mineral calcium. When calcium supplies dwindle, levels of a hormone called calcitrol go up, with a corresponding negative impact on fat burning. Calcitriol switches off mechanisms that break down fat and activates those that produce it. So you need dairy foods in your diet, not only for the calcium they provide, but also to support fat metabolism.

7. Choose from healthy fats. Enjoy a tablespoon a day of high-response cost, high-yield fats or oils, or, if the fat is a reduced-calorie product, have two tablespoons a day. Healthy fats are a hunger suppressor. No nuts or seeds are allowed in this stage, since it is too easy to go overboard on these foods.

8. Drink eight to ten glasses of pure water daily. Although you can enjoy a variety of non-caloric beverages, water is your best choice. Drinking too little water leads to dehydration, a state of imbalance that can slow down your metabolism.

9. Eat allowable foods (see below) only from the high-response cost, high-yield food lists. Use the food guide to familiarize yourself with these foods.

10. Do not stay in Stage 1 for more than 14 days, although you may return to this stage if your weight has reached a plateau.

FOODS TO EAT ON THE RAPID START PLAN: HIGH-RESPONSE COST, HIGH-YIELD FOODS

Proteins*

Eggs	Fish	Meat (lean cuts)	Poultry (no skin)	Protein Substitutes**	Shellfish
Hard-boiled	Bass	Beef	Chicken breast	Beans	Clams
Poached	Bluefish	Lamb	Chicken, minced lean	Lentils	Crab
Soft-boiled	Flounder	Pork	Cornish game hen	Soy-based and vegetarian foods	Lobster
Scrambled	Grouper	Veal	Turkey breast	Textured vegetable protein	Mussels
	Haddock				
			Turkey, minced lean	Tempeh	Oysters
	Halibut		Turkey sausage, lean	Tofu	Scallops
	Saithe or coley				Shrimp or prawns
	Salmon				
	Sea perch				
	Swordfish				
	Trout				
	Tune				
	Basically any fish				

*For more protein choices, refer to the appropriate sections in the high-response cost, high-yield section of the food guide.

**If you are a vegetarian, these foods can be used as your protein serving at meals.

Carbohydrates

Fruits (Raw)	Non-Starchy Vegetables	Starchy Carbohydrates
Apple	Alfalfa sprouts	*Vegetables:*
Apricot	Artichokes	Beans
Banana	Artichoke hearts	Corn
Blackberries	Asparagus	Lentils
Blueberries	Aubergines	Potato
Cherries	Bamboo shoots	Pumpkin
Grapefruit	Batavian endive	Squash, winter
Grapes	Beans, green or yellow	Sweet potato
Kiwifruit	Bean sprouts	Yams
Lemon	Beetroot	*Wholegrains:*
Lime	Beetroot greens	Amaranth
Mango	Broccoli	Barley
Melon	Brussels sprouts	Bulgur wheat
Nectarine	Cabbage	High-fibre cereals*
Orange	Carrots, raw	Millet
Papaya	Cauliflower	Oat bran, cooked
Peach	Celery, raw	Oatmeal
Pear	Chicory	Quinoa
Pineapple	Courgettes	Rice, brown or wild
Plum	Cucumbers	
Raspberries	Endive	
Strawberries	Kale	
Tangerine	Leeks	
Watermelon	Lettuce	
	Mushrooms	

* These include any cold cereal that contains more than 5 grams of fibre per serving. Refer to the section titled 'Cereals' on pages 178 to 179 of the guide.

Fruits (Raw)	Non-Starchy Vegetables (cont.)	Starchy Carbohydrates
	Mustard greens	
	Okra, cooked	
	Onions	
	Parsley	
	Parsnips	
	Peas	
	Peppers, all varieties	
	Rocket	
	Shallots	
	Spinach	
	Spring greens	
	Squash, summer	
	Swede	
	Tomatoes	
	Turnips	
	Turnip tops	
	Watercress	

Fats

Groundnut oil

Linseed oil

Olive oil

Rapeseed oil

Safflower oil

Salad dressings or mayonnaise, reduced fat

Sesame oil

Soft margarine (avoid products that list hydrogenated fats or partially hydrogenated fats on label)

Sunflower oil

Vegetable oils (non-hydrogenated)

Other Rapid Start Foods

Low-Fat Dairy (Milk and Milk Products)	Non-caloric Liquids and Beverages	Condiments
Cheese, reduced fat	Bouillon or broth, fat-free	Gelatin, sugar-free
Cottage cheese, low-fat	Diet sodas	Herbs and spices
Milk:	Coffee, brewed or instant	Horseradish
Buttermilk, reduced fat	Soda water	Ketchup (1 tablespoon)
Non-fat milk, reconstituted from instant with water	Tea	Mustard
Semi-skimmed milk	Tea, herbal	Sugar substitutes (aspartame, sucralose)
Skimmed milk	Water, bottled or tap	Taco sauce (3 tablespoons)
Soya milk		
Yogurt, sugar-free		Vinegar, all varieties

How to Build Your Meals from the Rapid Start Lists

Constructing your meal plans from these lists is simple and straightforward, but I've made it easier for you by including two weeks of Rapid Start Menus in the next chapter. So that you get headed in the right direction now, here is an overview of the plan, broken down to the daily level of what to eat and when to eat it.

Breakfast
1 protein serving
1 starchy carbohydrate*
1 fruit
1 low-fat dairy
1 non-caloric beverage

* Men: Add a starchy carbohydrate at lunch.

Lunch

 1 protein serving
 2 non-starchy vegetables
 1 fruit
 1 low-fat dairy
 1 non-caloric beverage

Dinner

 1 protein serving
 2 non-starchy vegetables
 1 fat
 1 non-caloric beverage

Snacks

 Fruit (if not eaten with a meal)
 Low-fat dairy (if not eaten with a meal)
 Raw vegetables

Structured in this manner, your meals might look something like this:

- A sample breakfast might consist of a scrambled egg, high-fibre cereal, skimmed milk, and half a grapefruit.

- A sample lunch might consist of tuna; a generous salad of fresh lettuce and tomatoes with a reduced-fat salad dressing; and a ripe, juicy peach for dessert.

- A sample dinner might consist of roast beef, green beans, and steamed yellow squash, with low-fat, sugar-free fruit yogurt for dessert.

Using the Rapid Start Plan, you have a strategy in place to generate immediate weight loss – and create positive momentum for sustained losses towards your goal and on through to maintaining your weight loss. This is a chance to get things flowing your way so you can make some real progress. Once you have successfully completed 14 days of the Rapid Start Plan, you are now ready to move on to Stage 2.

STAGE 2:
THE HIGH-RESPONSE COST, HIGH-YIELD WEIGHT LOSS PLAN

Nutritionally, you get to switch gears and eat additional amounts of high-response cost, high-yield foods in Stage 2, including extra choices in the categories of vegetables, fruits, starchy carbohydrates, healthy fats, and condiments. In addition to the foods listed in the Rapid Start Plan, the specific foods you may reintroduce in Stage 2 include:

Fruits: fruit juices (unsweetened), frozen fruits (unsweetened), and fruits canned in juice or packed in water.

Non-starchy vegetables: canned non-starchy vegetables.

Soups: all soups listed in the high-response cost, high-yield section of the guide (pages 276–283). Soups make an excellent prelude to a meal. If you eat soup, you will feel full, and you will tend to eat less at your meals.

Wholegrains: all cereals from the high-response cost, high-yield food lists; wholegrain breads and biscuits; wholewheat and spinach pasta; all starchy carbohydrates listed in the high-response cost, high-yield sections of the food guide (pages 284–357).

Fats: nuts and seeds; reduced-fat peanut butter; any fat listed in the high-response cost, high-yield section of the food guide (pages 262–265).

Condiments: all condiments listed in the high-response cost, high-yield section of the guide. Don't go overboard on condiments; use them sparingly and in the amounts listed in the guide.

Thus, in Stage 2, you can select from any and all of the high-response cost, high-yield foods listed in the guide. This stage gives you more nutritional leeway than the Rapid Start Plan does, and you should stay with it until you reach your get-real weight.

Stage 2 creates greater metabolic control so that your body uses more calories for energy rather than for fat storage. This is because the foods you will eat are low in sugar and refined carbohydrates, as opposed to high-fat, high-sugar foods, which tend to instigate weight gain when eaten in excess. By avoiding the wrong kind of carbohydrates, namely sugary, processed foods, you gain a tremendous edge in managing your weight.

Here are important guidelines for following the High-Response Cost, High-Yield Weight Loss Plan:

1. Continue to eat three regular meals a day (breakfast, lunch, and dinner), as well as two daily snacks.

2. Continue to eat protein at each of your main meals because of its positive effect on metabolism and appetite suppression.

3. Eat unlimited amounts of non-starchy vegetables (at least four or more servings of these vegetables, including salad vegetables, broccoli, cauliflower, green beans,

and spinach) daily. Don't stuff yourself; just eat until you feel satisfied. Choose from raw, or cooked from fresh or frozen, or canned. You may select from any and all of the non-starchy vegetables listed on pages 288 to 357 of the guide.

4. Increase your intake of starchy carbohydrates to two servings a day if you are a woman; three servings if you are a man.

5. Eat two servings of fruit daily. Remember, you can now choose from fruit juice (unsweetened), frozen fruit (unsweetened), or fruit packed in water or canned in its own juice. For a complete list, refer to pages 224 to 243 of the guide. But remember: for hunger suppression, fibre, and overall nutritional yield, it is preferable to select fresh fruits.

6. Eat two servings of low-fat dairy foods daily.

7. Choose from healthy, high-response cost fats, in the amounts specified: 1 tablespoon of oil, fats, or salad dressing; or 2 tablespoons of reduced-fat fats. Other allowable fats include nuts and seeds; these are listed on pages 262 to 265 of the guide, along with their correct serving size.

8. Drink 8 to 10 glasses of pure water daily.

9. Eat food only from the high-response cost, high-yield food lists. There is a huge variety of these foods so, again, consult the food guide frequently to familiarize yourself with them.

10. Stay on this plan until you reach your get-real weight. If you reach a plateau or need to restart the food plan, you may go back on the Rapid Start Plan for no more than 14 days.

How to Build Your Meals from the Food Guide Lists

To plan your meals in this stage, follow the template below and use the food lists in the guide:

Breakfast

1 protein serving
1 starchy carbohydrate*
1 serving of fruit juice
1 low-fat dairy product
1 non-caloric beverage

Lunch

1 protein serving
2 non-starchy vegetables
1 starchy carbohydrate
1 fruit
1 low-fat dairy product
1 non-caloric beverage

Dinner

1 protein serving
2 or more non-starchy vegetables
1 fat
1 non-caloric beverage

* Men: Add a starchy carbohydrate at lunch or dinner.

Snacks

Fruit (if not eaten with a meal)
Low-fat dairy product (if not eaten with a meal)
Raw vegetables

By way of example, your Stage 2 meals might look something like this:

- A sample breakfast might consist of turkey bacon, wholegrain toast, skimmed milk, and orange juice.

- A sample lunch might consist of vegetable soup, wholewheat biscuits, roast chicken, and fruit cocktail (water-packed) for dessert.

- A sample dinner might consist of grilled salmon, stewed tomatoes, a large tossed salad with low-fat dressing, and very low fat, sugar-free fruit yogurt for dessert.

Stage 2 is very 'livable', and you'll find twenty-one days of menus in the next chapter. These menus include a variety of foods and nutrients that are normally excluded on typical diets – foods that naturally promote positive changes in eating behaviour. These foods are mostly 'hunger suppressors' that help control your hunger to avert physiologically based cravings that you normally experience on restrictive diets. By following this plan, you will normalize your eating patterns, so that chaotic, mindless eating will become a thing of the past.

How Much to Eat: Portion Guidelines

The next important question that now must be answered is: exactly how much should you eat each day of various types of foods?

You should refer to the high-response cost, high-yield food lists beginning on page 150 to determine serving sizes of allowable foods for all three stages of the food plan.

If you do not like the idea of weighing and measuring, however, what I recommend is a system of portion management that frees you from the obsessive need constantly to handle measuring utensils and food scales all day long. All you have to do is picture portions of food relative to the size of your hand, or to other everyday items. For example:

Food	Portion Size
Meat, fish, or poultry	The palm of your hand, your computer mouse, or a deck of cards
Vegetables	
Raw	Your fist
Cooked	Your hand when cupped
Starchy carbohydrates	
Cereal and cooked grains	Your hand when cupped
Serving of bread	1 slice or size of a computer disk
Bagel	½ bagel
Muffin	½ muffin
American-style muffin	1 cake case
Savoury biscuits	Refer to number of biscuits listed in the food guide.
Pulses and other starchy vegetables	Your hand when cupped

Fruit

Raw piece	Tennis ball
Canned (water or juice), or frozen	Your hand when cupped
Berries (raw or frozen), raw chopped fruit	Your fist

Dairy foods

Milk and yogurt	Your fist
Cottage cheese	Your hand when cupped
Cheese	A pair of dice
Sandwich cheese	1 slice or size of a computer disk

Fats

1 tablespoon of fats, oils, salad dressings, or nuts and seeds	Your thumb to the first joint, a teabag, or a walnut

STAGE 3:
ULTIMATE MAINTENANCE

When you reach your get-real weight, you have crossed the finishing line. But this is not the end of the race. You must continue to manage your weight and place a high priority on keeping it off. Stage 3 – Ultimate Maintenance – is about keeping your weight under control for a lifetime. So don't quit until you've gone the distance. If you stop short now, you'll throw out all the hard work you've done so far. Do what it takes to maintain your weight, and you'll keep your momentum going in the direction of permanent weight loss.

When you are nutritionally maintaining and managing your weight, the good news is that you can eat slightly more food, provided you stay active and exercise on a very regular basis.

This plan liberalizes the number of servings you may eat, mainly from the high-response cost, high-yield food lists. As your guide in this regard, simply use the following serving allotments to assist you in your food planning; and post it on your refrigerator door:

- Protein and protein substitutes: 3 servings
- Non-starchy vegetables: as many as you like (don't skimp here)
- Starchy carbohydrates: 3 to 4 servings
- Fruits: 3 to 4 servings
- Low-fat dairy products: 2 to 3 servings
- Healthy fats: 1 to 2 servings

As a resource to help you, please refer to the sample Ultimate Maintenance menus provided in the next chapter. I've provided you with a week's worth of menus, consisting of 1,800 to 2,000 calories a day. You do not have to eat exactly as these menus specify; simply use them to direct your own food planning. But please take them seriously, along with all the other tools and techniques you are using to create the level of health you want and deserve.

When following the Ultimate Maintenance Plan, you must continue to exercise a degree of self-control over your eating. While no food is really off-limits, you must learn to refuse those foods you don't handle well and choose better ones. Don't eat a food that is a problem for you, because it may trigger a full-blown binge. As you follow this maintenance plan, please stay flexible. If you want to eat cake and ice cream at your child's birthday party, then, by all means, have it. But don't obsess over it and feel guilty. Obsessing over what to eat and what not to eat will only sabotage your maintenance efforts, making it more difficult to maintain your weight loss.

Your life should allow for some occasional treats, as long as you keep from bingeing or returning to a pattern of free-for-all eating.

Tools for Maintenance

Before leaving this chapter, let me be straight with you: the vast majority of people who eventually reach their target weight do not retain that goal. Did you know that there are just as many people trying to lose weight as there are people who are considered obese? The rate of obesity and the number of 'dieters' in America are climbing in parallel!

It's like this: you have a long history of learned and over-learned behaviours – in the way you eat, the way you think, the way you feel, and the way you act – so overlearned, in fact, that they have become second-nature habits to which you instinctually drift when under stress or pressure, or whenever you're not actively managing your weight, your health, and your life with a great degree of awareness and programming. Second-nature habits do not change quickly. That's why there is so much truth in the familiar saying *Old habits die hard*.

But STOP right here: this does not have to be true for you. If you have applied seven keys to your life, you now know something about why you eat and why you are overweight, and what you can do about it. Because knowledge is power, you have the wherewithal to get on the right track and head in a different direction.

When you maintain your weight, there is still a lot of work ahead. It takes effort, action, and commitment to shake free of your past negative programming. There is still a part of you that is comfortable in these old ways of being and doing, and it is that part of you that perhaps doesn't want things to change and will put up a good fight to resist it.

Having reached your goal weight, you may feel that you can handle things now and that you can let down your guard. But as I have often stated, *weight is managed, not cured*. You must never relax your watchfulness over your thoughts, feelings, and actions. Your guiding objective must always be to manage your weight, and indeed, your overall health, with a keen sense of alertness.

As you prepare to go forward into the future, let me encourage you to look back at the considerable work you did in *The Ultimate Weight Solution*. It's perfectly acceptable and, in fact, a good idea to 're-audit' your internal dialogue, emotional eating, stress, environment, nutrition habits, exercise, and support level. Maybe it helps to re-examine yourself in these areas in two, four, six months, or a year or more from now.

For right now, I'd like you to push to express yourself in specific terms: how and why it is important to you to maintain your weight loss. Perhaps because you reduced your intake of low-response cost foods and now eat more wholesome, high-response cost foods *in the amount your body needs for optimum functioning*, you love the physical and mental stamina you now enjoy. Maybe you realize that for you to keep your weight off, you must maintain certain good habits such as eating three structured meals a day, not skipping breakfast, planning ahead for what you will eat, and not eating food right out of its package. Maybe you now see the value of checking the number of calories or the correct serving sizes of food if you are unsure about what or how much to eat. Or possibly you recognize that staying active keeps you fit and makes you feel younger, more energetic, and less tempted to choose foods that would tear down this new-found physical vitality.

All of these sorts of descriptions should be expressed in what I call *Your Maintenance Management Formula*. This can serve as a written reminder of what you have personally learned about losing weight so that if your weight should ever start inching upwards again, you have a written, detailed description of what has helped you. This description, or formula, can also help you prepare in advance for various danger zones, or barriers, that lie in wait, so that you know how to handle them and then hang on to what you have worked so hard to achieve.

Let's start writing your maintenance management formula right now. All you have to do is fill out the sheet below by responding to the questions provided. Be detailed and thorough in your answers.

My Personal Maintenance Management Formula

Write five positive statements about why you like being at your get-real weight:

1. _____

2. _____

3. _____

4. _____

5. _____

Write a short paragraph below describing how it feels to have pulled this off:

_____

_____

_____

_____

_____

List five reasons why you do not return to being overweight:

1. _____

2. _____

3. _____

4. _____

5. _____

Make a list of the behaviours that have worked well for you. Use as much space as you need. This is an important opportunity to remind yourself of the programming that has helped you. (These behaviours might include not eating too fast, not eating while watching TV, eating more fruits and vegetables, selecting low-fat foods, or refusing to eat sugary foods; or this list could include habits such as exercising, keeping junk food out of your house, using incompatible substitutes to fight off eating urges and impulses, or practising positive, rational self-talk. If you need reminding, reread the relevant-to-you parts of *The Ultimate Weight Solution*.)

1. _____

2. _____

3. _____

4. _____

5. _____

6. _____

7. _____

8. _____

9. _____

10. _____

11. _____

12. _____

13. _____

14. _____

15. _____

16. _____

17. _____

18. _____

19. _____

20. _____

Make a list of what you see as your greatest barriers to maintaining your weight. Maybe these are bingeing when you are under stress or feeling fatigued. Perhaps you still think of yourself as overweight and unworthy, which puts you at a very high risk of regaining the fat you never psychologically shed. Or possibly you think you will relax your effort and slide back into some poor eating or exercise habits. Be specific and as concrete as you can when describing what you see as your toughest barriers up ahead.

1. _____

2. _____

3. _____

4. _____

5. _____

6. _____

7. _____

8. _____

9. _____

10. _____

For each barrier you identified and described, write a strategy or strategies for how you will overcome it. (If you want to, skip ahead and read through the next chapter – it contains some very effective strategies for weight loss and for weight maintenance – then come back here when you're finished.) Map out how you will handle this barrier in a rational, manageable fashion, without making foolish choices. Don't let yourself off the hook here. This is an important part of advanced planning so that you will not be hijacked by situations in your life.

1. _____

2. _____

3. _____

4. _____

5. _____

6. _____

7. _____

8. _____

9. _____

10. _____

Describe how you plan to 'self-monitor' your weight, and how often, from here on out to make sure that it is not creeping upwards again. Failure to self-monitor is one of the top reasons why people allow their weight to pile back on. Will you weigh yourself once a week? Will you measure your waistline? Will you check how your clothes fit, and whether they're getting too snug again in places? In the space below, write down how you will self-monitor, and how often.

Method(s) of self-monitoring:

_____

Frequency of self-monitoring:

_____

You should give yourself an acceptable weight-gain range, say five pounds or so, that you will not let yourself exceed. But if your weight does exceed that range, you must take action. What exactly will you do if your weight gets out of bounds? Get back on your calorie-controlled food plan? Start keeping your personalized food journal again? Reread and apply the seven keys? Work on more effective and meaningful accountability? Ramp up your exercise programme? In the space below, describe some specific steps that you will have to take to regain control (draw from what helped you before).

Steps for dealing with weight gain:

_____

_____

By answering the questions above and doing this work, you now have a working formula of exactly what you need to do in order to manage your weight for the long haul. Understand that once you create a proactive plan like this, you take a crucial step towards maintaining your focus and momentum and you pave the way for more success.

THREE

The Ultimate Weight Solution Menus

To make meal planning easy and workable for you, I've included several menu plans for all three stages: 14 days of Rapid Start menus; 21 days of High-Response Cost, High-Yield Weight Loss Plan menus; and 7 days of Ultimate Maintenance menus. There is also a sample vegetarian menu at the end of this chapter if you require help in figuring out such a food plan.

Initially, you might be more comfortable following a prescribed menu because it removes so much of the iffiness involved in meal planning and helps ease the transition into new ways of eating. With these menus, remember to refer to the food guide for serving sizes, or rely on the portion management guidelines I discussed in the previous chapter.

STAGE 1:
THE RAPID START PLAN:
14 DAYS OF SAMPLE MENUS

The Rapid Start menus supply an average of 1,100 to 1,200 calories a day, with approximately 30 per cent of those calories from protein, 45 per cent from carbohydrates, and 25 per cent from fat. On average, the menus furnish 30 grams of fibre a day. These menus are also low in sugar, sodium, saturated fat, and cholesterol.

Day 1

Breakfast
1 serving high-fibre cereal (e.g., All-Bran)
1 cup skimmed or soya milk
1 egg, scrambled (or two egg whites, scrambled)
Strawberries (or other seasonal fruit)
Coffee or tea

Snack
Pear

Lunch
Water-packed tuna with one sliced tomato served on a generous bed of lettuce, chopped green peppers, radishes, and other salad vegetables
2 tablespoons low-calorie Italian salad dressing

Snack
 1 cup low-fat, sugar-free plain yogurt mixed with
  1 tablespoon sugar-free apricot preserves

Dinner
 Roast chicken breast
 Asparagus spears, steamed or boiled
 Summer squash (crookneck), steamed or boiled

Day 2

Breakfast
 Grilled lean bacon, 2 rashers
 Oat bran cereal, cooked
 ½ grapefruit
 Coffee or tea

Snack
 Banana smoothie: 1 frozen banana blended with 1 cup
  skimmed or soya milk and artificial sweetener (optional)

Lunch
 Mediterranean salad: ½ cup chickpeas on generous bed of
  mixed greens and chopped salad vegetables
 1 tablespoon olive oil mixed with balsamic vinegar to taste

Snack
 1 cup low-fat, sugar-free yogurt (any flavour)

Dinner
 Grilled salmon
 Broccoli, steamed or boiled
 Carrots, cooked

Day 3

Breakfast

   Lean ham, 2 slices

   Sugar-free muesli mixed with 1 cup low-fat, sugar-free
      yogurt (any flavour)

   Orange

   Coffee or tea

Snack

   Apple

Lunch

   Chicken Caesar salad: cubed grilled chicken breast,
      shredded romaine lettuce, with an assortment of other
      chopped salad vegetables, 2 tablespoons reduced-fat
      Caesar salad dressing

Snack

   ½ cup low-fat cottage cheese, with baby carrots and other
      cut-up raw vegetables

Dinner

   Beef tenderloin

   Green peas, boiled

   Cauliflower, steamed or boiled

Day 4

Breakfast

   1 egg, scrambled

   Oatmeal, cooked

   1 cup skimmed or soya milk

   Cantaloupe (or other seasonal fruit)

   Coffee or tea

Snack
> Fresh berries

Lunch
> Black bean chilli: ½ cup cooked black beans, 2 tablespoons
> salsa, 2 tablespoons chopped onions, ½ cup stewed
> tomatoes

Snack
> 1 cup low-fat, sugar-free yogurt (any flavour)

Dinner
> Roast turkey breast
> Brussels sprouts, steamed or boiled
> Tossed salad
> 2 tablespoons low-fat French salad dressing

Day 5

Breakfast
> 2 egg whites, scrambled
> 1 serving high-fibre cereal
> 1 cup skimmed or soya milk
> Raspberries (or other seasonal fruit)
> Coffee or tea

Snack
> Cut-up assorted raw vegetables
> 1 ounce reduced-fat Cheddar cheese

Lunch
> Grilled chicken breast
> Shredded cabbage tossed with 2 tablespoons low-fat salad
> dressing

Snack
   Pear

Dinner
   Roast Cornish game hen
   Carrots, cooked
   Kale, cooked

Day 6

Breakfast
   Turkey bacon, 2 rashers
   Oat bran cereal, cooked
   Nectarine or peach
   Coffee or tea

Snack
   1 cup low-fat, sugar-free yogurt (any flavour)

Lunch
   Grilled hamburger, extra lean
   Tossed salad
   2 tablespoons low-fat salad dressing
   1 cup grapes

Snack
   ½ cup low-fat cottage cheese with cut-up raw vegetables

Dinner
   Baked cod or other white fish
   French-style green beans, boiled
   Yellow squash, steamed or boiled

Day 7

Breakfast

  1 egg, scrambled
  Wholemeal or granary toast, 1 slice
  Honeydew melon
  Coffee or tea

Snack

  Apple

Lunch

  Cooked aubergine topped with ½ cup tomato sauce, ½ cup
    cubed tofu, and 1 ounce of reduced-fat mozzarella
    cheese
  Tossed salad with 1 tablespoon olive oil and balsamic
    vinegar

Snack

  1 cup plain low-fat, sugar-free yogurt with 1 tablespoon
    sugar-free strawberry preserves

Dinner

  Roast pork tenderloin
  Cabbage, boiled
  Okra slices, boiled

Day 8

Breakfast

  Grilled lean back bacon, 2 rashers
  1 serving high-fibre cereal

1 cup skimmed or soya milk
½ grapefruit
Coffee or tea

Snack
Sliced cucumbers dipped in ½ cup low-fat cottage
cheese

Lunch
Vegetarian lunch: ½ cup kidney beans topped with
2 tablespoons salsa
Globe artichoke, steamed, leaves dipped in 2 tablespoons
low-fat Italian dressing
Raw baby carrots

Snack
Pear

Dinner
Lean steak
Tomatoes, stewed
Cauliflower, steamed or boiled

Day 9

Breakfast
Turkey bacon, 2 rashers
Smoothie: blend 1 cup skimmed or soya milk with
berries
Coffee or tea

Snack
Apple

Lunch

Grilled hamburger, extra lean

Spinach salad: chopped fresh spinach, ½ cup white beans,
2 tablespoons chopped onion, 2 tablespoons chopped
red pepper, and 1 tablespoon olive oil with balsamic
vinegar to taste

Snack

1 cup low-fat, sugar-free yogurt (any flavour)

Dinner

Roast chicken breast

Sugar snap peas or French beans, boiled

Fresh tomato, sliced

Day 10

Breakfast

2 egg whites, scrambled

Shredded Wheat

1 cup skimmed or soya milk

Banana, sliced

Coffee or tea

Snack

Plum

Lunch

Three-bean salad: ¼ cup chickpeas, ¼ cup kidney beans,
½ cup cooked green beans, 2 tablespoons chopped
onion, 2 tablespoons chopped roasted red peppers, and
2 tablespoons low-fat Italian dressing – served on a bed
of romaine lettuce

Snack

    1 cup low-fat, sugar-free yogurt (any flavour)

Dinner

    Crab, white meat (canned or fresh)

    Mixed vegetables, steamed (broccoli, courgettes, yellow
       squash)

Day 11

Breakfast

    1 egg, poached

    Oatmeal, cooked

    Orange

    Coffee or tea

Snack

    Fruit smoothie: 1 cup skimmed or soya milk blended with
       berries, with artificial sweetener (optional)

Lunch

    Minced turkey, lean, grilled

    Grilled portabello or large field mushroom

    Fresh tomato, sliced, topped with 1 ounce reduced-fat feta
       cheese

Snack

    Cut-up raw vegetables

Dinner

    Grilled salmon

    Broccoli and cauliflower medley, steamed

    Tossed salad with 1 tablespoon olive oil

Day 12

Breakfast
Grilled lean back bacon, 2 rashers
1 serving high-fibre cereal
1 cup skimmed or soya milk
Raspberries (or other seasonal fruit)
Coffee or tea

Snack
Pear

Lunch
Spinach and prawn salad: cooked prawns, 2 tablespoons
chopped onion, 1 sliced tomato, raw spinach, and
2 tablespoons low-fat mayonnaise

Snack
Cut-up raw vegetables dipped in ½ cup low-fat cottage
cheese

Dinner
Grilled sirloin steak
Broccoli, steamed
Yellow squash, steamed or boiled

Day 13

Breakfast
2 egg whites, scrambled
Porridge (or 1 serving high fibre cereal)
1 cup melon balls (or other seasonal fruit)
Coffee or tea

Snack
Orange

Lunch
Low-fat chef salad: 2 slices lean ham, 1 ounce
    reduced-fat Cheddar cheese, chopped lettuce and
    assorted cut-up salad vegetables, 2 tablespoons
    low-fat French dressing

Snack
1 cup low-fat, sugar-free yogurt (any flavour)

Dinner
Grilled tuna steak
Sugar snap peas, steamed or boiled
Asparagus, steamed or boiled

Day 14

Breakfast
Grilled lean back bacon, 2 rashers
1 serving high-fibre cereal
1 cup skimmed or soya milk
Sliced peaches
Coffee or tea

Snack
1 cup low-fat, sugar-free yogurt (any flavour)

Lunch
Grilled chicken breast
French-style green beans, boiled
Jacket potato, medium

Snack
  Banana

Dinner
  Roast beef
  Stewed tomatoes
  Tossed salad with 2 tablespoons low-fat blue cheese
    dressing

STAGE 2: THE HIGH-RESPONSE COST, HIGH-YIELD WEIGHT LOSS PLAN: 21 DAYS OF SAMPLE MENUS

The High-Response Cost, High-Yield Weight Loss menus supply an average of 1,200 calories a day, with approximately 30 per cent of those calories from protein, 47 per cent from carbohydrates, and 23 per cent from fat. On average, the menus furnish 25 to 30 grams of fibre a day and are low in sugar, sodium, saturated fat, and cholesterol.

Day 1

Breakfast
  1 egg, poached
  Oat bran, cooked
  1 cup skimmed or soya milk
  Banana
  Coffee or tea

Snack
  Apple

Lunch

Water-packed tuna

1 cup vegetable soup

Salad greens and sliced tomato with 2 tablespoons reduced-fat salad dressing

Wholemeal roll (medium)

Snack

1 cup low-fat, sugar-free yogurt (any flavour)

Dinner

Sirloin steak

Broccoli, steamed or boiled

Green beans, boiled

Day 2

Breakfast

1 egg, poached

1 slice multigrain bread

Raspberries (or other seasonal fresh fruit)

Coffee or tea

Snack

Skimmed or soya milk or low-fat, sugar-free yogurt (any flavour)

Lunch

Steamed prawns

Tossed salad with 1 tablespoon olive oil vinaigrette dressing

½ cup pineapple canned in water or natural juice

Snack

Cut-up raw vegetables dipped in ½ cup low-fat cottage
cheese

Dinner

Turkey breast
Stewed tomatoes
Summer squash, steamed
½ cup brown rice

Day 3

Breakfast

Grilled lean back bacon, 2 rashers
1 slice wholemeal or granary bread
½ grapefruit
Coffee or tea

Snack

1 cup low-fat, sugar-free yogurt (any flavour)

Lunch

1 cup vegetarian chilli
Cut-up raw vegetables dipped in 2 tablespoons reduced-fat
ranch salad dressing

Snack

Smoothie: skimmed or soya milk blended with frozen
strawberries

Dinner

Grilled chicken breast
Kale, boiled
½ cup mashed sweet potatoes

Day 4

Breakfast

    2 egg whites, scrambled
    American-style bran muffin
    1 cup orange juice
    Coffee or tea

Snack

    Low-fat, sugar-free coffee, vanilla, or lemon yogurt

Lunch

    Open-faced turkey sandwich: turkey breast, 1 slice
        reduced-fat Cheddar cheese, 1 slice wholemeal bread,
        lettuce and tomato slices, and 1 tablespoon reduced-fat
        mayonnaise

Snack

    Apple

Dinner

    Lean pork roast
    Spinach, steamed
    Tossed salad with 1 tablespoon reduced-fat salad dressing

Day 5

Breakfast

    Turkey ham (lean), 2 slices
    1 serving high-fibre cereal
    1 cup skimmed or soya milk
    Blueberries (or other seasonal fruit)
    Coffee or tea

Snack

Smoothie: skimmed or soya milk blended with frozen
unsweetened peaches

Lunch

Pitta sandwich: canned salmon, wholemeal pitta bread,
chopped celery, sliced tomato, and 1 tablespoon
reduced-fat mayonnaise

Raw carrots

Snack

1 cup low-sodium vegetable juice

Dinner

Roast Cornish game hen
Summer squash, steamed or boiled
Tossed salad with 1 tablespoon reduced-fat salad dressing

Day 6

Breakfast

2 egg whites, scrambled
1 serving high-fibre cereal
1 cup skimmed or soya milk
½ grapefruit
Coffee or tea

Snack

Diced mango (or other seasonal fruit)

Lunch

Greek salad: 1 ounce reduced-fat feta cheese, ½ cup
chickpeas, romaine lettuce, 2 tablespoons chopped

onion, 3 black olives (pitted), and
2 tablespoons reduced-fat Caesar salad dressing
Wholemeal bread (optional)

Snack

Raw baby carrots and other cut-up raw vegetables

Dinner

Grilled swordfish
Turnip tops, boiled
½ cup acorn squash, mashed

Day 7

Breakfast

Grilled lean back bacon, 2 rashers
½ small-diameter (6–8 cm/2.5"–3") wholemeal bagel
Cantaloupe
Coffee or tea

Snack

Smoothie: 1 cup skimmed or soya milk blended with a
frozen banana

Lunch

Steamed prawns, reduced-fat coleslaw and sliced tomato

Snack

Cut-up raw vegetables
1 ounce reduced-fat Cheddar cheese

Dinner

Lean minced beef

Mixed vegetables

Wholemeal pasta with low-fat tomato-based pasta sauce

Day 8

Breakfast

2 egg whites, scrambled

Oatmeal, cooked

1 cup skimmed or soya milk

1 cup sliced fresh peaches

Coffee or tea

Snack

Apple

1 cup low-fat, sugar-free yogurt (any flavour)

Lunch

Canned salmon, served on salad greens with 1 tomato,
sliced, and 2 tablespoons reduced-fat salad dressing

Snack

Fresh cut-up vegetables

Dinner

Roast pork tenderloin

Baked sweet potato, medium

Broccoli, steamed

Day 9

Breakfast
1 egg, poached
1 slice multigrain bread
Raspberries (or other seasonal fruit)
Coffee or tea

Snack
1 ounce reduced-fat cheese
Wholegrain biscuits

Lunch
Roast chicken
1 cup vegetable soup
½ cup fruit cocktail, packed in water or natural juice

Snack
1 cup low-sodium vegetable juice

Dinner
Roast turkey breast
Green peas
Stewed tomatoes

Day 10

Breakfast
Turkey bacon, 2 rashers
1 serving high-fibre cereal
1 cup skimmed or soya milk
½ grapefruit
Coffee or tea

Snack
> Pear

Lunch
> 1 cup vegetarian chilli
> Broccoli, steamed

Snack
> Cut-up raw vegetables with ½ cup low-fat cottage cheese

Dinner
> Chicken breast, grilled
> ½ cup sweetcorn, cooked
> Tossed salad with 1 tablespoon olive oil, mixed with
>   balsamic vinegar

Day 11

Breakfast
> Turkey ham (lean), 2 slices
> Smoothie: 1 cup skimmed or soya milk blended with
>   1 cup strawberries
> Coffee or tea

Snack
> 1 cup low-fat, sugar-free coffee, vanilla, or lemon yogurt

Lunch
> Tuna sandwich: water-packed tuna, 2 slices wholemeal
>   bread, lettuce, 2 slices tomato, and 1 tablespoon
>   reduced-fat mayonnaise
> Raw baby carrots

Snack

Apple

Dinner

Lamb loin roast

Cauliflower, steamed or boiled

Spinach, steamed or boiled

1½ teaspoons margarine for vegetables

Day 12

Breakfast

1 egg, hard-boiled

1 serving high-fibre cereal

1 cup skimmed or soya milk

Blueberries

Coffee or tea

Snack

Smoothie: soya milk blended with frozen banana

Lunch

Pitta sandwich: canned salmon, 1 wholemeal pitta bread,
2 tablespoons chopped celery, and 1 tablespoon
reduced-fat mayonnaise

1 cup tomato soup (condensed), prepared with water

Snack

Cut-up raw vegetables

Dinner

Roast Cornish game hen

Yellow squash, cooked

Tossed salad
1 tablespoon reduced-fat dressing

Day 13

Breakfast
2 egg whites, scrambled
American-style bran muffin
½ grapefruit
Coffee or tea

Snack
1 cup low-fat, sugar-free yogurt (any flavour)

Lunch
Greek salad: 1 ounce reduced-fat feta cheese, romaine
lettuce, ½ cup chickpeas, 2 tablespoons chopped onion,
3 black olives (pitted), and 2 tablespoons reduced-fat
Caesar salad dressing

Snack
Apple

Dinner
Grilled swordfish
½ cup mashed butternut squash
Turnip tops, steamed or boiled

Day 14

Breakfast
1 egg, poached
½ wholemeal muffin

Cantaloupe
Coffee or tea

Snack

1 ounce reduced-fat cheese
Rye crispbread

Lunch

Steamed prawns
Tossed salad, 2 tablespoons reduced-fat salad dressing

Snack

Grapes

Dinner

Reduced-carbohydrate 'spaghetti': meat sauce made with
lean minced beef and ½ cup low-fat tomato-based pasta
sauce served over cooked spaghetti squash
Steamed broccoli

Day 15

Breakfast

2 egg whites, scrambled
Sugar-free muesli mixed into 1 cup low-fat, sugar-free
yogurt (any flavour)
1 cup grapefruit juice
Coffee or tea

Snack

Pear

Lunch
 Turkey chef salad: reduced-fat turkey ham, 1 ounce
  reduced-fat Cheddar cheese, chopped tomato served
  over a generous bed of lettuce, with 2 tablespoons low-
  fat French dressing

Snack
 1 cup low-sodium vegetable juice

Dinner
 Grilled scallops
 ½ cup sweetcorn, cooked
 French-style green beans, steamed or boiled

Day 16

Breakfast
 1 egg, hard-boiled
 Smoothie: 1 cup skimmed or soya milk blended with frozen
  unsweetened blueberries
 Coffee or tea

Snack
 1 cup low-fat, sugar-free yogurt (any flavour)

Lunch
 Beef burger, extra lean, grilled
 1 wholemeal roll
 Cut-up raw vegetables
 2 tablespoons light ranch salad dressing, for vegetables
 Stewed tomatoes

Snack
> Banana

Dinner
> Roast turkey breast
> ½ cup brown rice
> Broccoli and cauliflower, steamed or boiled

Day 17

Breakfast
> French toast: 1 slice wholemeal bread, dipped in 1 egg
>   beaten with ¼ cup skimmed or soya milk, fried on
>   non-stick frying pan
> 2 tablespoons sugar-free syrup
> 1 cup orange juice
> Coffee or tea

Snack
> Smoothie: ¾ cup skimmed or soya milk blended with
>   1 frozen banana

Lunch
> Chicken Caesar salad: grilled chicken breast, romaine
>   lettuce, sliced tomato, and 2 tablespoons reduced-fat
>   Caesar salad dressing

Snack
> 1 cup low-fat, sugar-free yogurt (any flavour)

Dinner
> Baked ham, extra lean
> Baked sweet potato, medium
> Spring greens, boiled or steamed

Day 18

Breakfast

Grilled lean back bacon, 2 rashers
1 serving high-fibre cereal
1 cup skimmed or soya milk
Blueberries
Coffee or tea

Snack

1 cup low-sodium vegetable or tomato juice

Lunch

Reduced-fat burrito: ½ cup black beans, 1 corn tortilla,
2 tablespoons salsa, 3 tablespoons chopped onion, and
1 tablespoon jalapeño peppers
1 large tomato, sliced

Snack

½ cup fruit cocktail packed in water or natural juice
1 cup low-fat, sugar-free yogurt (any flavour)

Dinner

Grilled sirloin steak
Tossed salad with 1 tablespoon salad dressing
Mixed vegetables, steamed or boiled

Day 19

Breakfast

1 egg, scrambled
1 slice wholemeal or granary toast
1 cup grapefruit juice
Coffee or tea

Snack

Cut-up raw vegetables dipped in ½ cup low-fat cottage
cheese

Lunch

Chef salad: reduced-fat ham, 1 ounce reduced-fat Cheddar
cheese, salad greens, chopped red pepper, and 1
tablespoon olive oil, mixed with balsamic vinegar

Snack

Strawberries

Dinner

Grilled salmon
½ cup broad beans, boiled
Summer squash, steamed or boiled

Day 20

Breakfast

1 egg, poached
1 slice wholemeal toast
Banana
Coffee or tea

Snack

1 ounce reduced-fat cheese
Apple

Lunch

1 cup bean soup
Tossed salad
2 tablespoons reduced-fat salad dressing

Snack
1 cup low-fat, sugar-free yogurt (any flavour)

Dinner
Roast beef
½ cup mashed potatoes
Green beans, steamed or boiled
Courgettes, steamed or grilled

Day 21

Breakfast
Grilled lean back bacon, 2 rashers
Oatmeal, cooked
Blackberries (or other seasonal fruit)
Coffee or tea

Snack
1 cup low-fat, sugar-free yogurt (any flavour)

Lunch
Grilled chicken breast
Brussels sprouts, steamed or boiled
Carrots, boiled
1½ teaspoons margarine

Snack
½ cup pineapple packed in its own juice with ½ cup low-fat cottage cheese

Dinner
Baked ham, lean
Cabbage, boiled

½ acorn squash, baked
1½ teaspoons margarine

STAGE 3: ULTIMATE MAINTENANCE PLAN: 7 DAYS OF SAMPLE MENUS

With the Ultimate Maintenance Plan, you increase your calories to 1,800 to 2,000 calories a day, as well as add more servings of high-response cost, high-yield foods.

Day 1

Breakfast

1 egg, scrambled
1 bagel, with 1 tablespoon non-fat or very low fat cream or soft cheese
1 baked apple, medium
1 cup skimmed or soya milk
Coffee or tea

Snack

Pear

Lunch

Sandwich: lean sliced turkey, ham or chicken, 1 tablespoon reduced-fat mayonnaise, slice of tomato and 2 lettuce leaves, and 2 slices wholegrain bread
½ cup baked beans
½ cup coleslaw

Snack
    1 cup low-fat, sugar-free yogurt (any flavour)
    Peach (or other seasonal fruit)

Dinner
    Sirloin steak
    Tossed salad
    1 tablespoon non-fat salad dressing
    Vegetable medley: broccoli, cauliflower, carrots, summer
        squash – boiled or steamed

Day 2

Breakfast
    Grilled lean back bacon, 2 rashers
    Sugar-free muesli
    1 slice fruit bread toast
    2 teaspoons low-sugar jelly
    Berries
    1 cup low-fat, sugar-free, fruit-flavoured yogurt (any flavour)
    Coffee or tea

Snack
    Apple

Lunch
    Tuna salad: water-packed tuna, one celery stalk (chopped),
        1 tablespoon sweet relish, 1 tablespoon mayonnaise,
        and quartered tomato, served on a large bed of lettuce
    1 serving of wholemeal crackers
    Orange

Snack

Smoothie: skimmed or soya milk blended with 1 cup frozen
    unsweetened strawberries

Dinner

Roast chicken breast
½ cup brown rice
Broccoli, steamed or boiled
Stewed tomatoes
Fruit cocktail, in natural juice

Day 3

Breakfast

Turkey bacon, 2 rashers
Oatmeal or other cooked wholegrain cereal
Banana
1 cup skimmed or soya milk
Coffee or tea

Snack

Nectarine or other seasonal fresh fruit

Lunch

Peanut butter sandwich: 2 tablespoons reduced-fat peanut
    butter and 2 slices wholegrain bread
1 cup vegetable soup
2 cups cut-up raw cauliflower and broccoli with cherry
    tomatoes
Peach

Snack
  1 cup low-fat, sugar-free, fruit-flavoured yogurt (any flavour)
  Orange

Dinner
  Grilled salmon
  ½ cup mashed sweet potatoes
  Tossed salad
  1 tablespoon non-fat salad dressing

Day 4

Breakfast
  1 egg, scrambled (or 2 egg whites, scrambled)
  1 slice wholemeal toast
  1 cup orange juice
  Coffee or tea

Snack
  Smoothie: 1 cup skimmed or soya milk blended with frozen
    unsweetened fruit

Lunch
  Roast chicken
  1 chopped tomato on a large bed of salad greens
  2 tablespoons reduced-fat French salad dressing
  1 serving of wholemeal crackers

Snack
  Apple

Dinner

    Pork loin roast

    Turnip tops, boiled

    ½ acorn squash, baked

    Green beans, boiled

    ½ cup unsweetened applesauce

Day 5

Breakfast

    2 egg whites, scrambled

    1 American-style bran muffin

    1 serving high-fibre cereal

    1 cup skimmed or soya milk

    ½ grapefruit

    Coffee or tea

Snack

    Dried fruit

    2 tablespoons dry roasted peanuts

Lunch

    Chef salad: lean ham, 1 tomato (chopped), salad greens,
        and 2 tablespoons reduced-fat French dressing

    1 wholemeal roll, medium

Snack

    Cut-up raw vegetables

    3 tablespoons non-fat vegetable dip

Dinner

    Roast turkey

    ½ cup mashed sweet potatoes

Mixed vegetables, steamed or boiled
½ cup frozen low-fat yogurt
Blueberries

Day 6

Breakfast

1 egg, poached
½ muffin
Fresh chopped fruit
1 cup low-fat, sugar-free, fruit-flavoured yogurt (any flavour)
Coffee or tea

Snack

1 cup low-sodium vegetable juice
1 slice reduced-fat cheese

Lunch

1 cup bean soup
Tossed salad
1 tablespoon salad dressing, any flavour
Wholemeal roll
Apple

Snack

3 cups air-popped popcorn
Orange

Dinner

Baked or grilled scallops
½ cup brown rice
Mixed vegetables, steamed or boiled
Sliced cooked beetroot

Day 7

Breakfast

    1 egg, cooked (or 2 egg whites, scrambled)
    1 slice fruit bread toast
    ½ cup pineapple chunks, in natural juice
    1 cup skimmed or soya milk
    Coffee or tea

Snack

    Orange

Lunch

    Grilled hamburger, lean
    1 wholemeal bun
    Garnishes: 1 slice onion, 1 slice tomato, 1 leaf lettuce
    2 teaspoons mustard, 2 teaspoons ketchup
    Cabbage, boiled

Dinner

    Baked ham
    ½ cup mashed potatoes
    Asparagus, steamed

SAMPLE VEGETARIAN MENU

If you are a vegetarian, servings of meat can be replaced with any of the following: ½ cup beans/pulses (such as kidney beans); ½ cup tofu (great in pasta recipes); veggie burgers or soya burgers (available as frozen); meatless or soya frankfurters; or foods such as soya bacon, soya ham, soya sausage, and texturized soya protein, which resembles minced beef (this can be used to replace minced beef in various recipes). To replace dairy, use soya milk and soya cheeses. Thus, a good weight-management menu for a strict vegetarian would look something like this:

Breakfast
    Soya bacon, 2 rashers
    1 serving high-fibre cereal
    1 cup soya milk
    1 fresh fruit

Snack
    Pieces of celery filled with 2 tablespoons reduced-fat
        peanut butter

Lunch
    Large vegetarian chef salad made with a variety of mixed
        greens and salad vegetables, 2 slices of soya ham
        (diced), 1 ounce of soya cheese (diced), and tossed with
        2 tablespoons of fat-free dressing

Snack
    Soya smoothie: blend one cup soya milk with 1 frozen
        banana, ¼ teaspoon vanilla, and some artificial
        sweetener

Dinner

Tofu pasta dish: ½ cup cooked wholewheat pasta, ½ cup low-fat tomato-based pasta sauce, with seasonings, and ½ cup tofu (crumbled over pasta)

1 cup of cooked mixed vegetables, Italian style

For more menus, please log on to www.drphil.com, where you'll have an opportunity to participate in online support communities and learn valuable guidelines on weight loss and weight maintenance.

FOUR

No-Fail
Solutions:
Food Strategies
for Success

For successful weight management, you must have in place particular plans for dealing with what you know will be the weakest spots in your efforts. Your particular weakness could be poor behavioural control, eating away from home, poor eating habits in general, splurging on holiday, or overeating in response to stress. For example, do you typically drop in front of the TV with a bag of crisps when you get home from work? In social situations, do you eat and drink far more than what is in keeping with your weight management goals? At restaurants, or on holiday, do you eat to your heart's content, without thinking about what this might do to your waistline?

Whatever your trouble spot is – and I'm sure you already know it – you need some strategies, skills, and solutions that will allow you to stop sabotaging yourself and your weight.

This chapter is designed to give you those skills, and help you consider ways in which you can begin to make each of them more of a daily element in your life. The more you try to apply these things, the more successful your weight management efforts will be. So start now. Here are more than a hundred different ways you can change what is going on in your day-to-day life, and change your weight in the process.

BEHAVIOURAL STRATEGIES

You may get tired of hearing it, but I'll never get tired of repeating it. When you choose the behaviour, you choose the consequences.

Much of your excess weight can be traced directly to specific behaviours that are driving your results. Before you get defensive and retreat into denial, make no mistake about the following. Whatever your weight, you set it up that way. This does not mean that you did it on purpose. Nevertheless, you are the responsible party. Until you reckon with this fact, you will have a difficult time getting your weight management efforts under control.

To bring this point into sharper focus, please take a good look at my 'hit list' of weight-gaining behaviours on pages 94 and 95. I want you to see that the things you do really stack up, calorie-wise and pound-wise. Also, note in the fourth column how much weight you can gain over the course of one year unless you stop these eating behaviours. When you realize how you've been sabotaging yourself, you can learn from your mistakes and begin to remove these behaviours as barriers to your success.

The good news is that you can choose differently from now

on. You can behave your way to success. The following are positive steps you can take to help eliminate negative eating behaviours:

- Replace bad habits with incompatible actions. When you examine your own eating habits, and you get real about the fact that they are perpetuating your weight problem, then you need to eliminate them; you need to break those bad habits. 'Break' is actually a misnomer, because we don't actually 'break' habits. In order to eliminate one habitual behaviour, you must replace it with a new behaviour that is *incompatible* with the one you want to eliminate. When you make a new habit incompatible with the old one, the bad one will gradually lose its grip over you, since the two habits cannot coexist at the same time. For example, it is virtually impossible to spoon ice cream out of the container if you are taking a shower. Taking a shower is incompatible with gorging on ice cream.

  One reason this plan of attack works so powerfully is that substituting an incompatible behaviour for a bad habit takes your mind off the habit you want to weaken. When you are at work on activities such as gardening, playing with your kids, meditating, or writing in your journal, your mind is usually not on food.

  So the trick is to enact one or more incompatible substitutes when you feel like overeating, or otherwise going off your food plan. These activities form a new cadre of coping tools that you can substitute for overeating. The more tools and activities you can plug into your day as coping strategies, the more likely you are to get the results you want.

HIT LIST OF WEIGHT-GAINING BEHAVIOURS

Eating Behaviour	Weekly Caloric Cost	Annual Caloric Cost	Potential Weight Gain Per Year (3,500 extra calories = 1 pound)
Eating second helpings (200 calories per helping) three times a week	600 extra calories a week	31,200 extra calories a year	9 pounds
Habitual overeating, every day, 380 extra calories a day	2,660 extra calories a week	138,320 extra calories a year	40 pounds
Eating a super-sized bagel (12 cm/4.5" diameter, 323 calories) three times a week, rather than having a small bagel (8 cm/3" diameter, 156 calories)	500 extra calories a week	26,000 extra calories a year	8 pounds
Eating Big Macs (or equivalent, 570 calories) twice a week, rather than choosing a small-sized hamburger (260 calories)	620 extra calories a week	32,240 extra calories a year	9 pounds
Eating one glazed doughnut (290 calories) every day at work during your coffee break	1,450 extra calories a week	75,400 extra calories a year	22 pounds
Drinking a cup of whole milk (150 calories) twice a day, rather than having skimmed milk (86 calories)	896 extra calories a week	46,600 extra calories a year	13 pounds
Drinking one regular fizzy drink a day (144 calories), rather than having a calorie-free one	1,008 extra calories a week	52,400 extra calories a year	15 pounds

Behaviour	Per week	Per year	Annual weight gain
Snacking on 15 to 20 crisps a day (150 calories)	1,050 extra calories a week	54,600 extra calories a year	16 pounds
Eating a bowl of regular ice cream (280 calories) five times a week, rather than having a bowl of non-fat frozen yogurt (160 calories)	600 extra calories a week	31,200 extra calories a year	9 pounds
Bingeing twice a week (1,000 to 3,000 calories per binge)	2,000 to 6,000 extra calories a week	104,000 to 312,000 extra calories a year	30 to 89 pounds
Eating out at a fast-food restaurant five times a week (56 extra calories per fast-food meal), compared to having a healthy meal prepared at home	280 extra calories a week	14,560 extra calories a year	4 pounds
Snacking while watching television, five hours a week (136 extra calories per snack)	680 extra calories a week	35,360 extra calories a year	10 pounds
Night-time eating, five episodes a week (270 calories per episode)	1,350 extra calories a week	70,200 extra calories a year	20 pounds
Drinking three beers at Happy Hour once a week (146 calories per beer)	438 extra calories a week	22,776 extra calories a year	7 pounds

The information in this chart is based on typical caloric counts of foods and beverages, as well as on scientific studies of the caloric cost of specific eating behaviours. Results may vary from person to person. Annual weight gain is based on calculating the estimated yearly caloric cost of each behaviour, then dividing by 3,500 calories (the number of additional calories it takes to gain one pound).

The chart below lists numerous activities that compete with eating and can be used as incompatible substitutes. Use this list or create one of your own to push yourself into action when the urge to overeat hits you.

INCOMPATIBLE SUBSTITUTES FOR OVEREATING

Activities for Fun and Enjoyment

Pursue a favourite hobby, or take up something new you'd like to learn.

Work on a craft.

Work in your garden.

Play a game with your kids or your friends.

Learn a new sport or game.

Visit your neighbours, or talk to a friend.

Write letters or send emails to friends or family.

Write in your journal.

Give yourself a manicure.

Go to a good movie, or rent a video.

Read your favourite magazine.

Read a good book.

Plan your next holiday.

Watch a sunrise or sunset.

Spend time with your children.

Activities for Relaxation

Do relaxation exercises such as deep breathing or yoga.

Go for a walk, jog, swim, or bike ride.

Head to the gym and work out.

Exercise to an exercise video.

Dance to some upbeat music.

Take a shower or a leisurely bath.

Have a massage.

Pamper yourself with a day of beauty at a day spa or salon.

Listen to music.

Sing along with your favourite music.

Engage in prayer or meditation.

Write a poem.

Take a short nap.

Take the day off and go on a day trip.

Activities You Must Do

Do housework.

Work on a home improvement project.

Pay your bills.

Balance your chequebook.

Rearrange the furniture in a room or two.

Wash your car.

Clean out your closets or your drawers.

Run errands.

Do all the things your dentist wants you to do – brush, floss, rinse with mouthwash.

Volunteer for a project, then follow through on your commitments.

Take your dog for a walk.

- Change your eating style. Certain eating behaviours can lead to weight gain. These include eating too fast, snacking while watching television, sampling food while cooking, and eating in several rooms in your home, among other habits. These and other habits are examples of *mindless eating,* in which you shovel in an enormous amount of calories in a very short period of time without even realizing it. What you must do is replace mindless eating with its incompatible substitute, *mindful eating,* in which you concentrate on what and how you are eating. Mindful eating helps prevent overeating and leads to constructive behavioural change. What follows are some specific strategies you can use to counter mindless eating with mindful eating.

If you are a fast eater who needs to slow down:

- After your food is placed in front of you, wait five minutes before you eat it.
- Place small mouthfuls of food on your fork or in your spoon.
- Completely swallow food from each mouthful before you add any more to your fork or spoon.
- Put your utensils down between bites.
- Use smaller utensils (try a cocktail fork, for example) – no soup spoons, ladles, or otherwise oversized tableware for shovelling in food.
- Consciously take time to taste, chew, and savour the food you eat.
- Stretch out your meals, making them last thirty minutes instead of five or ten minutes, to allow for a reduction in hunger. One way to do this is to take a five-minute break at about ten minutes into your meal.
- Take sips of water or other non-caloric beverages between bites.
- Introduce a one- or two-minute delay between courses.

If you have trouble patrolling your portions:

- Measure your food if you're afraid of overeating.
- If you don't have the patience to measure out your food, use plates, glasses, and bowls in the serving sizes you need.
- Use a smaller plate for your meals.
- Purchase single-serving foods.
- Try the divided plate method of portion control. Fill half your plate with non-starchy vegetables, one fourth of your plate with a starchy carbohydrate, and the remaining fourth with a lean protein.

If you have a habit of eating leftovers:

- Put away all the food involved in preparing a meal.
- Have the table cleared of serving plates.
- Leave the table after you've finished eating.
- Have someone else clean leftovers off the plates after meals.
- Ask your family to scrape their plates directly into the garbage disposal or bin after meals so that you won't be tempted to gorge on the leftovers.
- Leave some food on your plate.
- Purchase food in smaller packages or quantities so that you rarely have leftovers.

If you tend to eat while standing or while on the move:

- Localize your eating: select one area of your home – your dining room, breakfast nook, or some other area reserved only for eating – and eat *all* of your food at a designated table in that area. That includes regular meals, snacks, and beverages.

- Vow not to eat while driving in your car; standing in front of your open refrigerator; reading a book, magazine, or newspaper; sitting in your bed; or talking on the phone. In other words, do not pair other behaviours with eating. Doing so only distracts your attention from your eating behaviour, and you will lose all sense and awareness of how much you are consuming. If you are engaging in any of these behaviours while eating, you're not focused on your eating. This means you are not in control.
- Stop eating foods right out of their bags or packages.

If you sample food while cooking:
- Place a small portion of the food on a plate; sit down and taste it.
- Chew sugar-free gum while cooking.
- Minimize your time in the kitchen.
- Ask someone else in your family to prepare meals occasionally.

If your eating is chaotic and largely unplanned:
- Keep your personalized food diary. It is an effective tool for meal planning as well as a self-diagnostic tool for pinpointing small slips in your behaviour before they become big ones. It lets you review and learn from your behaviours.
- Change your routine so that your drive to and from work doesn't take you by bakeries, fast-food restaurants, or other tempting sources of food.
- Make food choices mindfully by asking yourself a simple question: 'Does this food or meal, in this

amount, contribute to my health and to effective weight control?' If the answer is no, if you are choosing to eat something, or too much of something, that does not support your goal of health and weight management, then you need to rethink your decision.

If you overeat at night:

- Brush your teeth in the evening after dinner to signal that you've finished eating for the night.
- Read a book or magazine prior to going to bed; or substitute any activity you can think of that is incompatible with eating.

If you watch television while snacking:

- Eat only in your designated eating place – at your kitchen or dining-room table.
- Eliminate all distractions while eating – including television (turn it off).
- Continue to keep problem foods out of your house, or else you'll indulge when an impulse to eat seizes you.

Mastering even one or two of the preceding bad behaviours will liberate you from counterproductive eating and dramatically reduce your weight. So if you want your weight to be lower than it has been in the past, get to work on these actions and disciplines. They will bring success.

Nutritional Strategies

Other areas for improvement may involve making some day-to-day tweaks in your nutrition and meal planning. Do you skip meals because you think you don't have enough time to eat? Do you go shopping without a list and end up filling your larder with foods you don't need? When you choose healthy foods, are you eating the same boring rabbit food, day after day, and now you're deep in a food rut that is causing you to rebel? You are about to find some extremely useful ways to help you create results that are better aligned with reaching your get-real weight. So let's put some more verbs in your sentences and some more action into your life with the following.

- Do not – I repeat, do not – skip breakfast. Your body requires refuelling after going eight to twelve hours without food. Not eating breakfast leads to cravings later and is a factor in overweight and obesity. If time is a problem in the morning: fix a breakfast shake or smoothie, made by blending fruit and low-fat milk; eat a bowl of packaged high-fibre cereal; or have a meal replacement bar or beverage, along with some fresh fruit.

- Expand your nutritional repertoire and try something new. Each week introduce into your diet at least one fruit or vegetable you've never touched in the past.

- Cook 'in bulk' on the weekends. Have cut-up vegetables ready for salads; mashed sweet potatoes ready for reheating; chilli that can be microwaved; or chicken breasts that can be warmed up.

- Shop for 'healthy' convenience foods, such as salad in a bag, so that you don't have to spend time chopping up salad vegetables.

- If you are in a hurry or too tired to cook and you must pop a packaged food into the microwave for a meal, at least serve it with a salad and fruit for dessert.

- Purchase more low-fat cooking gadgets – non-stick pots and pans, vegetable steamer, or rice cooker – to help you prepare more dishes that do not require the addition of fat.

- If you must help yourself to seconds, help yourself to vegetables.

- Cut the cocktails. Alcohol provides a triple whammy: it increases your appetite, lowers your inhibitions so you eat more, plus research shows that drinking alcohol will cause your body to store more calories as fat.

- Plan in advance when you will snack and what you will eat for that snack. This is far better – and safer – than unplanned snacking, for example, having a bag of crisps or a bowl of sweets that you mindlessly grab while watching TV or reading.

- Choose snacks from high-response cost, high-yield foods that supply good nutrition, rather than from nutritionally weak foods: a small American-style bran muffin instead of a pastry, an apple instead of biscuits, a glass of skimmed milk or soya milk instead of a soft drink.

- Take the same healthful snacks to work so that you won't be tempted by vending machine selections or fattening food brought in by your co-workers.

- Never eat any snack from its original container or package. Place it on a plate and eat your snack in a designated place.

- When food shopping:
  - Shop from a list, prepared when you are not hungry or stressed out.
  - Determine exactly what you need for a particular period of time, and don't overbuy.
  - Stick to the outer aisles where the fresh, additive-free foods are located. There's a logical reason for this placement: fresh foods require more frequent restocking and therefore must be situated as close to the outside shipping docks and stockrooms as possible.
  - Never go shopping when you're hungry. The entire supermarket, from the food aisles to the checkout queue, can tempt you to buy foods that you neither want nor need.
  - Assign someone else in your family the job of shopping on occasion in order to limit your exposure to food.

- Try not to use food as a reward when you've reached mile-markers on the way to your get-real weight. This undoes any good you've done to yourself and shifts into reverse any progress you've made towards your weight loss goals. Instead, reward yourself with a new outfit, a new pair of walking shoes, a trip to a day spa, a new CD or DVD, or a special book.

What you have just read about are small, manageable changes you can easily make in activities you do every day. If you get practical about making these changes, you will begin the process of reprogramming yourself to get in the shape you want to be in.

RESTAURANT STRATEGIES

For many of you, eating away from home, particularly at restaurants, is problematic. The key is to take some time to pre-plan for those situations and identify those things that could and should be the focus of your management efforts. When you decide to dine out:

- Select a restaurant that offers a variety of foods so that you can choose healthier menu items.

- Obtain a copy of the menu before going to a designated restaurant in order to decide ahead of time what you will order.

- Take control over the choice of restaurant. Go where you know you can order food that supports your weight control goals.

- Call the restaurant in question to determine whether they serve low-fat or low-calorie foods.

- Be assertive with the waitstaff; tell your server you want your food prepared without fats, oils, or sauces.

- Avoid all-you-can-eat and buffet-style restaurants, at least until you are less vulnerable to the sight of food. If you must go to a buffet-style restaurant, survey the entire buffet before you jump in the queue so that you can decide which selections are the healthiest and will support your weight control efforts. Use a smaller plate at buffet-style restaurants – either a salad plate or a dessert plate. Visit the food queue only once; don't give in to the lure of the all-you-can-eat deal. Opt to order from the menu (if available), rather than choose from the buffet.

- Avoid ordering complete dinners, which often include unneeded portions, and opt instead for à la carte selections, since they give you more control over what you eat.

- If you know you are going to eat out for dinner, plan to have a lighter lunch to help balance and control calories.

- Say 'no' to cocktails when dining out. Alcohol is high in sugar and calories, with the potential to contribute to weight gain. In addition, alcohol overstimulates your appetite and lowers your inhibitions about overeating.

- Ask the server to remove the bread basket after you've been served (hopefully your dinner companions will support you in this request). Removing the bread removes a huge temptation and source of extra calories.

- Curb your appetite by ordering a cup or bowl of broth-based soup, or a salad, prior to your meal.

- Stop sabotaging yourself with starters (other than a light soup or salad). The calorie counts of some of the most popular starters are through the roof. For example, fried onion rings = 2,000 calories; barbecued chicken wings = 1,000 calories.

- Order high-response cost main courses – those that take time and effort to eat. Some suggestions: peel-and-eat steamed prawns, steamed crab legs, artichokes, or a large dinner salad with dressing on the side.

- Get fluent in restaurant lingo. Sauces like béchamel, Béarnaise, gratin, and hollandaise are synonyms for high fat and high cholesterol. *Sautéd* usually means cooked in butter. *Fried* is a red flag, since all fried food is loaded with fat and calories. So are gravy and cream sauces, since these are high in fat, cholesterol, and calories.

- Be clear, specific, and *polite* when making requests of your server. Simply state: 'I'd like my chicken grilled dry, without butter, oil, or margarine.'

- If you're feeling that your resolve is weak, have someone order for you. Make sure that someone is in your
  circle of support and will order a healthy, low-calorie
  main course for you.

- When ordering a salad, ask for dressing on the side,
  order half the dressing, or request no dressing at all
  (opt for lemon or vinegar instead).

- Consider sharing a main course with your dining
  companion, particularly if the restaurant is known for
  over-sizing or super-sizing its portions.

- When ordering beef, stick to lower-fat cuts. These
  include sirloin, flank steak, and tenderloin. Lower-fat
  pork and veal selections include pork chops, pork
  loin, veal chops, and roast veal. (High-fat meats
  include prime rib, diced steak, minced lamb or pork,
  spareribs, and pork sausages.)

- Trim all visible fat from your meat.

- For poultry, order skinless chicken or turkey, while
  generally staying away from goose or duck (which
  tend to be higher in fat).

- Stick to main courses that are cooked by simple
  methods, such as grilling, baking, steaming, roasting,
  or braising. Fancier dishes such as casseroles are very
  likely to contain elevated levels of fat, calories, cholesterol, and sodium.

- Your best bets for breakfast at restaurants include hot and cold cereals (unsugared), fresh fruit, unsweetened fruit juices (small size), skimmed milk, artificially sweetened low-fat yogurt, or eggs, scrambled egg whites, or scrambled egg substitutes. Avoid large or jumbo American-style muffins (they're loaded with fat, sugar, and calories); and pancakes, waffles, or French toast (which are usually prepared on a greased griddle).

- For lunch, avoid the urge to choose quick-to-eat low-response cost foods when time is at a premium (as it usually is during the lunch hour). Stick to salads with dressing on the side, while staying away from potato salad, macaroni salad, and coleslaw, which are usually made with a ton of mayonnaise. Sandwiches made with wholemeal bread or pitta bread and white-meat poultry or lean roast beef are preferable to cheeseburgers or sandwiches prepared with high-fat meats like salami sliced or pastrami.

- Practise salad bar smarts. Stick to leafy greens and lettuces, fresh vegetables, and reduced-fat dressing. Don't spoon dressing over your salad; instead, pour it into a small bowl so that you can use a small, designated amount on your salad.

- Be aware of fattening additives lurking in certain salad bar items. Three-bean salad, for example, is high in sugar. Cottage cheese at some salad bars is of the whole-milk variety and therefore high in fat. So are prepared salads (again – potato salad, macaroni salad, and coleslaw), as well as shredded cheese. Bacon bits, gherkins, and olives are high in sodium.

- A lot of restaurants will make up a vegetable plate for you if you ask them.

- Practise your behavioural eating-style skills not just at home, but also at restaurants: after your food is placed in front of you, wait five minutes before you eat it. Place small mouthfuls of food on your fork or in your spoon. Pause between bites and put your knife and fork down. Completely swallow food from each mouthful before you add any more to your fork or spoon. Consciously take time to taste, chew, and savour the food you eat. Take sips of water or other non-caloric beverages between bites.

- For dessert, choose fresh fruit, fruit salad, or sorbet (which is usually fat-free but higher in sugar).

- Don't feel guilty about leaving food on your plate. Do it!

- Ask the server not to bring the dessert trolley to your table.

- Do an audit of your 'dining-out frequency'. Count up how many times a week you eat out at restaurants. If your frequency is excessive – such as seven or more times – then you need to rethink your dining-out habits. People generally tend to eat more food when dining out. Plus, there is a lot of hidden fat and sugar in menu items you'd think were low-cal, so you may be sabotaging yourself unnecessarily here. Make a commitment to eat out no more than once or twice a week (such as on Friday evenings to celebrate the end of the work week), or on special occasions such as a birthday or anniversary. Make eating out an event, not an everyday occurrence.

TRAVEL AND HOLIDAY STRATEGIES

Travelling and taking holidays can be difficult too, but try to exert the same control in your choice-making that you would do at home or when eating out. If you're having difficulty in these areas, here are some strategies worth enacting:

- If you are flying, you don't have to settle for the typical airline food. If travelling by air, call the airline ahead of time (usually twenty-four hours) to request a special meal. Airlines can usually accommodate diabetic, vegetarian, low-fat, low-calorie, and low-sodium meals. You can make such requests practically anywhere, even on cruises, as long as you give the food preparation personnel plenty of notice.

- If the circumstances are such that you simply cannot control your choices, take it easy and eat smaller portions.

- If possible, take your own food to guarantee some control over what you eat while travelling or on holiday.

- Never travel on an empty stomach. This makes you less likely to cave in to food cues, such as fast-food vendors at airports. Eat a healthy, filling meal before you start your trip. If feasible, consider packing light and healthful snack foods, such as fresh or dried fruits, or cut-up vegetables.

- Self-monitor your food intake while away from home, using your personalized food diary and this food guide to help you stay the course. Pack both of these items.

- If your alcohol consumption tends to increase while on holiday, devise strategies to compensate, such as ordering soda water, diet drinks, or other non-alcoholic but low-calorie beverages.

- Do not take a holiday from your workouts. Stay with your regular exercise programme by walking, using hotel exercise facilities, or purchasing a week's membership at a local gym. During layovers, walk briskly around the airport for exercise. Exercising will burn off extra calories, plus help relieve the stress that is so often associated with travelling.

SOCIAL STRATEGIES

Staying the course during special occasions such as holidays, parties, or celebrations can be a challenge unless you have plans in place to deal with the circumstances. Make a deal with yourself that you will try at least one or two of these the next time you are confronted with a social situation that makes it tempting to overeat or disregard your food plan:

- Plan ahead. On days when you'll be attending parties or get-togethers, consume fewer calories by eating a light breakfast and lunch. 'Bank', or save, most of your calories for later on.

- Continue to self-monitor during the holidays by writing down what you eat and how many calories you consume in your personalized food diary. Research suggests that people who self-monitor their food intake can and will lose weight during the holidays.

- Consider a 'pre-diet'. Try losing two or three pounds prior to the holidays to give yourself some room to move up the scales.

- Eat something light before you go to a party in order to avoid arriving too hungry. If you let yourself get too hungry, your stomach and your eyes will make your food choices for you, instead of your brain.

- Concentrate more on people and conversation at parties, and less on the food or drinks.

- Make the most nutritious choices possible at parties or gatherings: fresh fruits, raw vegetables, wholegrain crackers, or lean proteins.

- If you are the host or hostess, there is no rule of hospitality that says you must serve fattening food to your guests. Try concocting lower-fat foods by altering recipes and using low-fat substitutes for high-fat ingredients. For example, you can replace all or part of the sour cream in dip recipes with plain low-fat yogurt. High-fat cheeses can be replaced by lower-fat products. You can also use reduced quantities of salt, sugar, and other sweeteners in recipes.

- Deal effectively with saboteurs. Your friends and family may present the biggest challenges to changes you want to make, especially at family get-togethers and celebrations. Sometimes friends and family won't take no for an answer and want to push food at you. In cases like this, try replies like, 'No thanks, I just ate.' 'Can't have that. Doctor's orders.' 'Can you wrap it for me?' (Then toss it once you get home.) 'Better not. An extra helping means an extra workout this week.' 'I'd love to, but I've got that class reunion coming up.'

  Guard against feeling guilty for focusing attention on yourself and standing up for yourself. It's okay to make time for yourself so that you can reach your goals. You must take care of yourself before you can take care of others, and now is the time to do that.

- Take control of the social situation. If you're invited to an event where mostly low-response cost, low-yield foods will be served, graciously ask the host or hostess if you can bring some of your own food. Or be direct. Explain why you are not eating certain foods. You may be surprised at how some people may start supporting you when you stand up for yourself like this.

If, after all your planning and good intentions, you do overindulge, don't go on a guilt trip. Guilt is a useless emotion that only weakens your resolve to manage your weight successfully. Get over it and move on.

STRESS-EATING STRATEGIES

Never in your life will you be without stress – problems, challenges, and difficult moments that are simply a part of living. You know that if things are going well at work, for example, you can count on conflict at home, or vice versa. There is rarely a time in your life when all is at peace and balanced. That's not good or bad; it is simply the ebb and flow of how life works. To be alive means to experience stress.

With stressful situations comes the potential for overeating as a way to escape anxiety and pressure. If you're someone who struggles with your weight, then I'm willing to bet that you medicate with food as a stress reliever a good deal of the time, abusing food because it provides comfort and consolation when you are worried, irritated, annoyed, lonely, bored, or depressed.

Stress – particularly when it is prolonged and unresolved – provokes weight-sustaining physiological changes in your body. When you are under stress, your body releases stress hormones that automatically stimulate your appetite and set off cravings, prompting you to eat huge quantities of fattening foods. These stress hormones trigger other bodily changes that may result in greater fat distribution around your waist. Overeating as a way to cope with stress may prove fatal to your weight-management efforts. You've got to step up and out of this behaviour. Take a moment now to consider some of the following strategies:

- Be accountable for how you react to stress. One of my life laws states that *there is no reality; only perception*. What this means is that you are accountable for how you respond to everything in your life. Whether it's an infuriating phone call, a lost opportunity, or a person who has treated you poorly, your response to that event creates your experience.

  But behind that response is a perception – the way you interpret or assign meaning to what you are experiencing. If your response (your interpretation) to a stressor is typically negative, pessimistic, or gloom-and-doom, you are creating an experience for yourself that is self-defeating and infinitely more stress-provoking. On the other hand, if you interpret the situation more positively, or realistically, you won't be so likely to become unglued, fall apart, or go into panic mode.

  When it comes to how you see things, you do have choices. You choose the reactions that create your level of stress. You have the power to choose your own perceptions and your own reactions; start choosing differently, with more clarity, more confidence, and more self-control. If you shake up your belief system and test your typical perceptions and reactions to events, rather than blindly or habitually holding on to them, the freshness of your new perspective can be startling. The freshness of your perspective can keep you from falling apart and resorting to food when the going gets tough. (Reading key 2, Healing Feelings, in *The Ultimate Weight Solution* will give you additional insights for managing the stress in your life and the emotions it produces.)

- Take a problem-solving approach to stress. Confront head-on whatever is wrong in your life and do something about it. If you don't, if you let these problems go unchallenged, you will pay the price and set yourself up for further physical and mental breakdown. The push to resolve the stress-provoking situation must come from you. You can either sit around and stew about the stressful situation or you can make the choice to be self-directed, take action, and adopt a solutional approach to your life.

- Nourish your body with healthy alternatives. There are nutritious foods that will induce the same calming effect as high-sugar comfort foods, but without the unpleasant side effects. Among the most effective anxiety-management foods are fresh fruits, vegetables, and wholegrains. Specifically, these foods are natural carbohydrates, which release serotonin, a brain chemical that lifts and improves your mood. Green leafy vegetables such as spinach and romaine lettuce are bursting with a vitamin called folic acid, a mood-balancing nutrient. Other good-mood foods include fish and unprocessed turkey. Fish, in particular, is a food that has been linked to a lower incidence of depression because of the brain-healthy fats it contains.

  The point is, for emotional comfort from food, you have to build certain foods into your food plan to help you normalize your mood for the day. This is nutritional knowledge that you can put to use on a day-to-day basis. Rather than sabotage your body's true needs, you can support them with high-nourishment foods.

• Practise relaxation. If you're stressed out and treat yourself to a plate of biscuits or a bag of sweets because you 'deserve it', get real. There are other ways to treat yourself and restore calm without resorting to a food binge. That's why you must carve out time in your life for tension-reducing activities. I suspect that if you habitually overeat in reaction to stress, then you have no clue as to how to relax without a food binge. You are more accustomed to putting something fattening in your mouth to get relief rather than using non-food activities to calm yourself down.

These alternatives include, but are not limited to, exercising (a powerful stress reliever!), performing relaxation exercises, and listening to music. According to most research, these activities work directly on your nervous system by releasing endorphins, the brain's natural tranquillizers, to produce a state of reduced anxiety and a feeling of calm. These activities are natural, non-chemical, and inexpensive relaxants.

There's no good reason for you to experience any nutritional backsliding when you have strategies in place to handle it. When these situations arise, as you know they will, you won't panic and start eating everything in sight. You will simply say to yourself, 'This is the very thing I knew would happen, and I know how to deal with it. I won't panic, and I won't give in just because I am encountering normal challenges of day-to-day life. I am in control.'

As you manage your weight, never lose sight of the stakes

involved. Your stakes are your health, your emotional well-being, your hopes and dreams, and the quality of your entire life. If you choose to bail out on managing your weight, be prepared to be another casualty of poor lifestyle decisions and choices.

Each day of progress you make, each action you take, has a positive effect. Trust in your ability to do it, and never forget that small and subtle changes in what you do are moving you in the right direction.

FIVE

How to Use the Food Guide

We all have room to improve the quality of our health in general and our diets in particular. So often, we need the right tools and the right knowledge to guide us. Now you've come to the part of this book where you will find valuable reference material on food that relates primarily to its effect on your weight and to your ability to manage it. This section provides information on the nutritional content of high-response, high-yield foods – the type of food you should eat – and low-response, low-yield foods – the type of food you should limit or avoid.

If you are familiar with *The Ultimate Weight Solution: The 7 Keys to Weight Loss Freedom*, you know that I am not a fan of counting calories, calculating carbohydrate or fat grams, or multiplying nutrient percentages. What I do advocate, however, in any change or improvement, is accountability – a way to check yourself to make sure that you are progressing steadily towards your get-real weight. Accountability can come in the form of a person in your circle of support to whom you commit to make periodic reports on what you plan to do, and it can come in the form of an informational tool like this book. This guide provides a measure of accountability by furnishing information to help you choose which foods are best for healthy weight management.

Without the accountability that this fundamental information provides, you are apt to con yourself about certain foods, thinking that they may not be so fattening after all. Then you're left wondering why you're not shedding weight as steadily as you wish or meeting your get-real weight goal. So consider this information carefully. The more you learn about the nutritional content of these foods, the better equipped you will be to make positive changes and increase your chances of living vigorously throughout your entire life.

ACCESSING FOODS IN THE GUIDE

I have organized *The Ultimate Weight Solution Food Guide* in such a way as to make it as convenient as possible for you to locate, look up, and access foods you want to include in your meal planning. In the pages that follow, the guide is organized into my two broad classifications of foods: *High-Response Cost, High-Yield Foods* and *Low-Response Cost, Low-Yield Foods*, each with a huge listing of individual foods. Under each classification, foods are alphabetized into categories such as Beef, Beverages, Cheese, Cereals, and so forth. Within those categories, individual foods in their many variations and options are listed for you in alphabetical order as well. This breakdown of foods is intended to make it easy to find the foods you want to look up.

Let's say, for example, that you want information on apples, a high-response cost, high-yield fruit. Check the table of contents, where you'll find an alphabetized listing of food categories, and go to 'fruits' under the high-response cost, high-yield listing. Turn to the page where the fruit listings begin and go to the 'a's. Fruits appear alphabetically, so it is easy to locate 'apples'. Under 'apples', you will find nutrient information for various types of apples, including raw, and peeled or unpeeled.

Now let's move on to talking about the nutrient information in my food guide. Each food entry lists the following information in this order: food name, serving size, calories, and the amount of each of the following (in grams or milligrams): protein, carbohydrate, total fat, saturated fat, cholesterol, fibre, sugar, and sodium. The information targeted in this guide is relevant for lifetime weight control. Keeping an eye on these nutrients can have a hugely significant impact on your weight and on the overall health of your body. Here is an explanation of each piece of nutrient information and why it is important.

Serving Size

The Ultimate Weight Solution Food Guide defines for you exactly what healthy, sensible portions should be, so you should use this information to determine the size and amount of your portions at meals.

Unfortunately, the world of food has changed – and changed drastically. Over the past twenty years, the portion sizes of foods we normally eat, both at home and at restaurants, have been increasing exponentially. You know I'm right, but as proof, a number of nutritional studies published in scientific journals in recent years have turned the rock over regarding this trend, only to reveal some rather alarming findings. Consider these statistics from America:

- Hamburgers have 'grown' from 5.7 ounces to 7 ounces (an increase of 97 calories).
- Mexican-style foods such as burritos and tacos have increased from 6.3 ounces to 8 ounces (an additional 133 calories).
- The classic recipe for American Toll House chocolate chip cookies from a 1949 cookbook yields 100 cookies; today, the same recipe in an updated, revised cookbook yields 60 cookies. This means the cookies are almost twice as big if you follow the recipe in the modern edition of the cookbook.
- A 16-ounce Coke is today considered 'small', yet supplies 202 calories – a huge amount for a beverage.
- Car manufacturers now install larger cup holders in new models in order to accommodate these super-sized drinks.

I could go on, but here is the problem with all of this as I see it: the food and restaurant industries, in particular, have so oversized food and meals that, as a food-consuming society, we have been conditioned over time to think that 'large', 'giant', and 'monster' sizes are the norm. What is astonishing is that we no longer recognize which amounts of food are correct and appropriate for our weight and our level of physical activity. We have let ourselves get brainwashed!

Most people can no longer differentiate between a normal-sized serving and a super-sized one. We've started to look at a cheeseburger as a cheeseburger, never mind that it is giant or gargantuan-sized.

Super-sized starts to look right-sized, often with terrible health consequences, one of which is obesity in children and adults. It is simply no coincidence that the super-sizing of food portions has paralleled the super-sizing of Americans, that is, the alarming rise in obesity.

The larger the portion, the more calories it has in it. Furthermore, it has been proven, time and time again in research, that large portions encourage people to eat more. It is simply a fact of eating behaviour that people will eat what is put in front of them. If more food is there, you will eat more food.

As consumers, we value a greater quantity of food and drink for a lower price – a value that the food industry is more than willing to provide. We also buy on impulse, and the food industry capitalizes on this behaviour. So when a server asks you, 'Do you want to super-size that?', go on alert. One survey of fast-food restaurants discovered that upgrading, or super-sizing, a meal at a burger restaurant provided 1,380 more calories for only 58 cents more. That's a great value – until you realize what it is doing to your waistline.

You and your family are being reeled in by these billion-dollar industries. I'm calling on you to stop taking the bait. Don't be lured by these deals. Know the costs to your weight and to your health. If you continue to cave in to impulse buying and the lure of the meal deal, then you're setting yourself up for more years of being overweight. It's about you deciding whether you are going to be baited for the rest of your life, waiting to get hooked. You control what you buy or don't buy; you control where you eat and what you eat when you get there. Like it or not, a lot of cause and effect is in your hands. The more knowledge you have about what's going on in the world around you, the more power you have to control the outcomes in your life.

If this guide is to be of any value to you, you must commit to referencing its serving sizes when you plan meals or go out to eat. You won't have to do this forever, just long enough to relearn what 'sensible' means in relation to 'super-sized'.

If you understand that portion sizes can doom your weight control efforts, then you've got the battle half won. You'll stop eating more than you need and more than you want because you have figured it out. In short, you get it.

Calories

As I have already emphasized, I am not in favour of counting or memorizing calories, because for many people trying to lose weight, this fuels obsessions with food and dieting. What's more, most people have neither the time nor the patience to count calories. Managing your portion sizes is a better way to go, because it automatically curbs your caloric intake.

Even so, I feel that it is important at least to be aware of the caloric content of certain foods – particularly low-response, low-yield foods, since many of these foods contain a rather shocking level of calories. (Did you know, for example, that 16 ounces of a flavoured coffee may contain nearly 400 calories?) You may think you know the calorie count of every food, but then again, you may not. Most people still need a refresher course in calories, mainly because of super-sizing and the fact that servings today are larger and contain far more calories than most people think.

What is well known, though, is that eating a certain number of calories each day will help you lose or maintain your weight. When you eat more calories than your body requires metabolically or can burn off in activity, you will store the surplus as fat. Eat fewer calories than your body needs, and your body will start burning fat for energy.

The magic number in weight management is 3,500 – the number of calories to create one pound of fat. For perspective, 3,500 calories of food equals about fifteen 1.5-ounce chocolate bars or fifty-seven slices of white bread. Eat that many chocolate bars or that many slices of bread, in addition to your normal three squares a day, and you will gain a pound of fat.

Reducing calories is the chief determinant of weight loss. You can do this by decreasing the number of calories you consume and/or by increasing the amount of exercise you do. For most people, a balanced plan of 1,200 to 1,500 calories a day, without the wholesale restriction of entire food groups, is effective for shedding excess pounds. If you are unsure of the calorie count of some foods, or how many calories you consume on a day-to-day basis, you can use this food guide to look them up and keep yourself accountable.

Protein

Protein is the nutritional equivalent of a handyman, absolutely essential for the repair and maintenance of your body, fixing up and renewing it on a day-to-day basis. You need protein to make hormones, disease-fighting antibodies, and muscle tissue – and to some extent, to provide your body with energy. Protein is typically found in fish, poultry, meat, and dairy products. Grain products and vegetables (particularly beans and pulses) supply some protein too.

In this food guide, most of the serving sizes for animal proteins such as meat, fish, and poultry are given in 4-ounce servings to deliver a slightly higher amount of protein in your diet. Protein has important metabolic effects on weight loss and thus plays a critically important, yet sometimes uncredited, role in healthy weight management. When provided at slightly higher levels in your diet, protein helps step up metabolic activity for greater fat-loss potential. As a hunger suppressor, protein is also filling; having some at each meal keeps your appetite in check. Furthermore, you will regain less weight during maintenance if you continue to eat higher-protein meals after you have lost weight. Because of its metabolic benefits, sufficient protein in your diet improves your ability to maintain your weight loss.

For effective weight loss, protein should comprise approximately one-fourth to one-third of your total daily calories, or 25 to 33 per cent. On a 1,200-calorie diet, that translates to 300 to 400 protein calories a day, or 75 to 100 grams; on a 1,500-calorie diet, 375 to 500 calories a day, or 94 to 125 grams.

Carbohydrates

These energy foods have been much maligned, accused of being excess calories from the major fat promoters. In truth, though, it is largely excess calories from the processed and refined variety of carbohydrates (like those found in white bread, cake, and snack foods) that is causing so much of the trouble. Loaded with added sugar and fat, processed carbohydrates tend to raise your blood sugar, and since what goes up must come down, there is a corresponding drop in blood sugar after a couple of hours. This state of low blood sugar results in food cravings. So when you eat refined, processed carbohydrates, your hunger returns rapidly – which is why such foods are hunger drivers. Plus, in response to that surge in blood sugar, your body releases the hormone insulin, which encourages the storage of calories as fat. By avoiding these foods in favour of natural, higher-fibre carbohydrates (fruits, vegetables, and wholegrains), you gain a tremendous edge in managing your weight.

Ideally, a diet in which 40 to 45 per cent of your daily calories come from healthy, high-fibre sources of carbohydrates will produce a good rate of weight loss. (That equates to 480 to 540 calories, or 120 to 135 grams, on a 1,200-calorie diet; 600 to 675 calories, or 150 to 169 grams, on a 1,500-calorie diet.)

The optimal number of grams of carbohydrates per day to drive weight loss has not yet been nailed down conclusively; however, you can lose weight efficiently with 120 to 175 grams a day, without dipping below 100 grams and sacrificing your physical and mental energy as a result.

The grams of carbohydrates represented in the food guide are the total grams of carbohydrates. Although listed separately in the guide, the grams of sugar and fibre are counted as part of total carbohydrates.

Total Fat

You need some fat in your diet, largely because fat supplies nutrients called 'fatty acids'. These vital components of fat drive a number of important chemical activities in your body, including the production of energy, the protection of cell membranes, and the absorption of vitamins A, D, E, and K (collectively known as the fat-soluble vitamins).

From a weight-control standpoint, fat has some very specific advantages. As a hunger suppressor, it is slow to break down and thus makes you feel full even after protein and carbohydrates have left your stomach. Fat also prompts your intestinal walls to release a special hormone that curbs the appetite and may help prevent overeating.

Clearly, fat is good for your body – but not in excess. The surplus calories you eat from fat are more likely to be stored as body fat than calories from either protein or carbohydrates, and nutritional research bears this out. Okay, so what about all those diets that let you slather butter and mayonnaise all over your food? Please understand something about such diets: they still reduce calories, and calorie reduction is the number one factor, the common denominator, that drives weight loss. When calories are over and above your metabolic needs, you'll get fat, and when those extra calories are mostly from fat, you'll probably get fatter. Of course, there is no question that a lower-fat diet helps normalize total cholesterol: LDL cholesterol, HDL cholesterol, and triglycerides – all the various blood fats that figure into the health of your cardiovascular system.*

Generally, the recommendation for good health is to curtail your fat intake to 30 per cent or less of your total daily calories. Using the chart below, find the average number of calories you eat daily, then look to see how many grams of fat should comprise your maximum intake in order to keep your daily fat calories at around 30 per cent.

Average Daily Calories	Fat
1,200	40 grams
1,500	50 grams
1,800	60 grams
2,000	67 grams
2,200	73 grams
2,400	80 grams

In the food guide, you will find the total fat content (in grams) of high-response, high-yield foods, as well as of low-response, low-yield foods. If you wish, use this information to add up the number of grams of fat you eat throughout the day. It is good planning to choose foods lower in total fat. By

*LDL (low density lipoprotein) cholesterol, often called 'bad' cholesterol, is the sort that clogs the arteries increasing the risk of heart disease. HDL (high density lipoprotein) cholesterol is the form in which cholesterol is removed from the body – which is why it is referred to as 'good' cholesterol.

US government labelling standards, a food product considered 'low-fat' contains less than 3 grams of fat per 100 gram serving, and 'fat-free', less than 0.15 grams.

You do not have to become an obsessive fat gram counter, however. Populating your diet with enough vegetables and some fruits and some wholegrains automatically ensures a lower-fat diet, eliminating the need to fixate on fat grams.

Saturated Fats

Part of the total fat in foods is saturated fat, found mostly in animal products. It is smart, and indeed a good idea, to pay attention to the amount of saturated fat in certain foods because of its health implications. Saturated fats raise total cholesterol and levels of LDL cholesterol by interfering with the liver's ability to remove cholesterol from your blood. In addition, saturated fats make your cells insensitive to the hormone insulin (technically termed 'insulin resistance'), whose job it is to clear excess sugar from your bloodstream. As a consequence, cells have trouble removing excess sugar from your blood.

As a general rule, foods that are high in saturated fats also tend to be high in a dangerous type of fat known as trans fats, found mostly in hard margarine, vegetable shortening, and many processed foods. If a food label reads 'hydrogenated' or 'partially hydrogenated oil', this indicates the presence of trans fats. Trans fats push cholesterol levels up and have other detrimental effects on your health.

Saturated fats should make up no more than 10 per cent of your total daily calories. Your saturated fat gram maximum, based on your daily average calories, is listed in the chart below.

Average Daily Calories	Saturated Fat
1,200	13 grams
1,500	17 grams
1,800	20 grams
2,000	22 grams
2,200	24 grams
2,400	27 grams

If you'd rather not have to tally up saturated fat grams, the following list provides guidelines on how to lower your saturated fat intake automatically.

How to Slash Fat and Saturated Fat

- Scrap the fatty meat and replace it with leaner cuts, fish, poultry, or vegetable-based proteins such as beans or lentils.

- Trim the fat off meat prior to cooking it.

- Cook meat or poultry on a rack so that the fat will drain off.

- Remove the skin from chicken, turkey, or other poultry prior to cooking (poultry skin is very high in fat).

- Avoid buying pre-basted turkey, which is sometimes injected with coconut oil (very high in saturated fat).

- Do not add oil to water while cooking pasta. (The addition of oil only prevents boilovers; the pasta doesn't need it.)

- Do not add butter, milk, or cream when making

mashed potatoes. Try skimmed milk, fat-free evaporated skimmed milk, or buttermilk instead.

- Be familiar with high saturated fat foods and avoid or limit them in your diet (refer to the chart below).

- Continue to use only low-fat or non-fat dairy products.

- Get friendly with trans-free margarines and spreads. Many of these are listed in the high-response cost, high-yield section of this guide.

- Avoid non-dairy creamers and non-dairy toppings. These are high in saturated fat from coconut or palm oils.

- Replace whole milk in recipes with its less fatty counterparts: skimmed milk, semi-skimmed milk, soya milk, evaporated skimmed or low-fat milk, or buttermilk.

- Sauté vegetables in broth or bouillon rather than in butter or margarine.

- Use 'yogurt cheese' in place of sour cream and high-fat dips. Spoon two cups of non-fat plain yogurt into a coffee filter; place the filter in a strainer that fits over a bowl, cover, and place in the refrigerator overnight. In the morning, you will have yogurt cheese, which can be mixed with herbs and used for dipping raw vegetables.

- Cut back on whole eggs, and instead use egg whites, which contain virtually no fat.

- For cooking, use a cooking spray rather than adding butter, margarine, or oil.

- An olive oil spray can add flavour to salads, vegetables, and chicken and fish dishes, but without the fat calories. The spray distributes a tiny bit of fat over a lot of food and can save you nearly 100 calories of fat.

- At the supermarket, look for low-fat alternatives to yogurt, cottage cheese, salad dressings, and mayonnaise.

- Slash the fat or oil in recipes by a third, or replace part of the fat with applesauce. You will not sacrifice flavour or texture.

Foods High in Saturated Fat

Bacon
Beef fat
Butter
Cheese
Chocolate
Cocoa butter
Coconut oil
Commercially baked goods
Cream
Cream cheese
Egg yolks
Fatty meats and poultry
Fried foods

Hydrogenated vegetable oil
Ice cream
Lard
Margarine
Milk, whole
Palm and palm kernel oil
Salami and other processed sliced meats
Shortening
Sour cream
Suet

When you're cutting back on saturated fats and trans fats, don't eliminate fats that are good for you. These include unsaturated fats, found in fish and vegetable oils. They can trigger healthy drops in triglycerides and bad cholesterol (LDL) in

WHEN A DOSE OF FAT IS DANGEROUS

High-fat meals can be inherently harmful. They step up the rate at which blood clots, and abnormal clotting is the instigator of most heart attacks. What's more, high-fat meals make your arteries less elastic, and this impedes blood flow through them.

If you want to protect yourself against this danger, try to make sure that your meals are mostly low-fat ones. What exactly constitutes a 'low-fat meal'? For women, this generally means a meal with 15 grams of fat or less (4 grams of saturated fat or less). This is based on a daily limit of 45 grams of total fat and 12 grams of saturated fat.

For men, this generally means a meal with 20 grams of fat or less (6 grams of saturated fat or less). This is based on a daily limit of 65 grams of total fat and 18 grams of saturated fat.

your blood, plus help your body handle blood sugar more efficiently. Other top-drawer fats that exert strong protection include olive oil, rapeseed oil, and flaxseed oil; all are useful and healthy additions to good nutrition.

In the food guide, you will find that fat content per serving is expressed as total fat/saturated fat. For example: for 4 ounces of roasted chicken breast, the entry is 4 grams/1 gram. Foods considered low in saturated fat contain less than 1 gram of this type of fat per serving.

Cholesterol

Cholesterol is a fat-like substance manufactured by your liver and provided in your diet through animal products such as eggs, meat, poultry, fish, dairy products, and lard. Only foods of animal origin contain cholesterol.

Eating foods with cholesterol can raise the cholesterol in your blood, but only to a small extent. As a general rule, about 15 per cent of the cholesterol in your blood comes from the food you eat, and the rest – 85 per cent – is manufactured by your body. In most people, the body maintains an equilibrium in response to dietary cholesterol. If you eat a lot of high-cholesterol foods, then your body will make less cholesterol, for example. What really hikes up your blood cholesterol, particularly LDL cholesterol, is eating too much saturated fat. So to reduce cholesterol in your blood, it is vital to slash the saturated fat in your diet.

There is a percentage of Americans – about 20 to 30 per cent – who are sensitive to dietary cholesterol, however. These people, along with anyone at risk for heart disease (if you're overweight, or have high blood pressure or elevated blood fats, you're at risk), should monitor their dietary cholesterol. The American Heart Association recommends 200 mil-

TOP 30 FOODS FOR CURBING CHOLESTEROL

These foods all contain a type of fibre known as soluble fibre, which has a cholesterol-lowering effect in the body, and may be good dietary choices for improving your blood cholesterol profile.

Non-starchy Vegetables
- Artichoke
- Turnip
- Brussels sprouts
- Cabbage
- Broccoli

Starchy Vegetables
- Sweet potato
- Acorn squash
- Potato with skin

Beans and Pulses
- Kidney beans
- Borlotti beans
- Butter beans
- Black beans
- Chickpeas
- Haricot beans

- Lentils
- Pinto beans
- Soya-based foods

Fruits
- Mango
- Figs, dried
- Kiwifruit
- Orange
- Plum

Cereals and Grains
- Oat bran
- Oatmeal
- Sultana Bran
- All-Bran
- Bran flakes
- Pearl barley

ligrams a day of dietary cholesterol for those with heart disease or its risk factors (overweight and obesity are risk factors), and 300 milligrams a day for the general population.

The food guide can make you accountable to yourself in this regard, since it lists the cholesterol content in food. A 'low cholesterol' food is one that contains 20 milligrams or less of cholesterol per serving.

Fibre

Fibre is the indigestible portion of plant foods that keeps our digestive system running smoothly. It also keeps you trim by promoting feelings of fullness, stabilizing your blood sugar, and keeping your hunger at bay. You're less likely to overeat at a single sitting if your meal is a high-fibre one.

Certain types of fibre, namely fibre from fruits and vegetables, have a modest calorie-curbing effect, too. Fibre pushes food through your digestive tract more rapidly. As a result, your body may not have enough time to absorb all the calories and fat that pass through and so they are excreted. Fewer calories are left to be stored as body fat. Scientific evidence suggests that if you follow a high-fibre, low-fat diet, as this plan suggests, you can lose three times more weight than if you followed a low-fat diet only.

Pulses (beans and lentils), fruits, vegetables, and wholegrains are among the foods most plentiful in fibre. You need between 25 and 35 grams a day of fibre for good health. Foods considered high in fibre contain at least 2.5 to 3 grams or more per serving. Fibre is one nutrient definitely worth counting.

A NOTE ON COUNTING FIBRE IN THE UK:

Since the early eighties, the UK food industry has used the Englyst method for determining the amount of fibre in a food while other EC countries and the USA use the American Association of Analytical Chemists (AOAC) method.

These two methods use different scales and therefore are not comparable; the AOAC method will, for many foods, give higher values for fibre compared to the Englyst method. **The fibre values in this book are calculated using the AOAC**

method. The UK recommended daily fibre intake is 18 grams for adults and this is based on the Englyst method. Using the AOAC method, the proposed benchmark is 24 grams.

However, it is essential that the two figures are not compared directly against each other. Looking ahead, the Food Standards Agency issued a notice in December 2000 to inform the food industry that the AOAC method would now be used in order to harmonise free trade. For more information on how the methods differ, please go to the British Nutrition Foundation website: www.nutrition.org.uk

COUNTING FIBRE

Here are some easy-to-remember ways for calculating fibre so that you reach at least 25 grams:

Foods with 6 grams or more
½ cup canned kidney beans, chickpeas, broad beans, or
  black beans
1 serving of All-Bran cereal

Foods with 4 to 5 grams
1 cup fresh berries (strawberries, blueberries, or raspberries)
1 pear with skin
1 serving dried fruit
1 serving bran flakes or Sultana Bran
1 cup cooked broccoli
1 medium sweet potato (baked with skin)

Foods with 2 to 3 grams
1 apple with skin
1 banana

1 orange
1 cup raw chopped vegetables
1 slice high-fibre bread
½ cup cooked grains (brown rice, wild rice, barley)
½ cup wholewheat pasta

Sugar

So many of you have failed to lose weight and keep it off because of sugar and sweets. If a hunk of your calories comes from sweet, sugar-laden food, it is likely that your natural

APPROXIMATE SUGAR CONTENT OF POPULAR FOODS*

Food	Teaspoons
Fortune cookie	1 teaspoon
Digestive biscuit	2 teaspoons
Oatmeal biscuit, fat-free	3 teaspoons
Vanilla ice cream, ½ cup	3 teaspoons
Sugar-coated breakfast cereal, 1 bowl	4 teaspoons
Cereal bar	5 teaspoons
Chocolate bar	5 teaspoons
Cranberry sauce, 1 slice	5½ teaspoons
Jelly, 1 bowl	6 teaspoons
Danish pastry	7 teaspoons
Yogurt, fruit-flavoured, low-fat, 8 ounces	7 teaspoons
Fizzy drink, cola, 12 ounces	10 teaspoons
Vanilla shake, fast-food, 20 ounces	12 teaspoons
Bottled fruit drink, 20 ounces	17 teaspoons

* Estimates were tabulated from USDA data and from food labels.

chemistry is almost constantly in a state of metabolic turmoil. Refined sugar (also called 'added sugar') and foods that contain it are digested quickly and they dump sugar into the bloodstream quite rapidly. In many people, this makes insulin levels spike upwards, causing calories to be converted into sustainable body fat rather than being burned for energy. It's not uncommon to experience more hunger and more cravings in the aftermath of this insulin response – all of which can lead to overeating.

Sugar and sweets can also be, for many people, as addictive as cigarettes, drugs, or alcohol, summoning up a loss of control that resembles the behaviour of addiction, and they can be just as difficult to give up. Physiologically, these foods excite the same circuits in your brain that are stimulated by pleasure-inducing drugs, delivering a mild and short-lived high.

If sugar is a problem for you, you have to acknowledge this fact and go about changing it. You cannot achieve a trim, fit body if you keep caving in to sugar cravings. Your body will just not cooperate. Failure to give up added sugar will create more trouble than you can ever imagine.

But the good news is that once you kick the sugar habit, your desire for sweets will probably diminish. If you avoid sweets, for even a few weeks, your taste buds will become deprogrammed from loving the taste of sugar, and you'll experience fewer cravings.

You need to recognize what the sabotaging effects of eating too much sugar are on your body and the role it plays in your weight. You also need to be aware of how much sugar there is in foods – which is why this food guide includes grams of sugar per serving in many of the foods listed. That way, you can start cutting back on sugar-added foods in order to get better control of your weight.

But what limits should you place on sugar consumption? There is no easy answer to that question, since recommended

DE-SUGAR YOUR DIET

- Use the food guide to track the sugar you consume during the day, since it can really mount up. Eating a bowl of frosted cold cereal, a can of cola, and a chocolate bar, for example, can add nearly 70 grams of sugar to your diet.

- Drink water, diet sodas, or herbal teas in place of sweetened fizzy drinks.

- Avoid sugary low-response cost, low-yield foods, such as sweets, biscuits, cakes, pies, pastries, and other sugary baked goods – even fat-free versions, which often contain as much sugar as their counterparts.

- Choose canned fruits that are packed in water or in their own juice.

- Get in the habit of having fresh fruit for dessert and snacks instead of having sweets. Eventually, your choice will shift from sweets to natural foods that will satisfy you in a big way.

- Avoid fruit drinks, beverages, and 'ades'; these products contain only 5 to 10 per cent real juice and are loaded with added sugar.

- Prepare your own fruit-flavoured yogurt by adding fresh or canned fruit to plain yogurt, or blend in sugar-free preserves or jam.

- Use artificial sweeteners, but use them in moderation.

levels for sugar intake have not been established. One prevailing recommendation is that you cap your intake of added sugar at 10 per cent or less of your total daily calories. For example:

Average Daily Calories	Added Sugar Maximums
1,200	30 grams
1,500	38 grams

1,800	45 grams
2,000	50 grams
2,200	55 grams
2,400	60 grams

Generally, each gram of sugar in a food comes from 4 teaspoons of sugar, although some of that sugar may come from natural sources if the food is a fruit, vegetable, or dairy product. 'Sugar-free' foods provide less than 0.3 gram of sugars per 100 gram or 100 ml serving. (Sugar-free does not mean carbohydrate-free.) If a food label says 'no sugar added', this means that no form of sugar has been put into the food during processing or packaging.

Be aware, too, that sugar in foods often comes disguised under other names on labels (see page 148 for an explanation of hidden sugars in foods), so you may be eating more added sugars than you think you are. For tips on reducing sugar in your diet, see the box on page 142.

You do not need to worry about the natural sugar in fruits, vegetables, and dairy products, however. This type of sugar comes wrapped up in vitamins, minerals, fibre, and antioxidants and is not the source of your excess pounds.

Sodium

Another food additive that is a potential health liability for some people is sodium. Foods in their natural state contain some sodium, a mineral that helps maintain normal water balance in the body and helps regulate the rhythm of your heart. Most sodium in our diets, however, comes in the form of sodium chloride, better known as 'table salt', that is added to food during processing. Many low-response cost, low-yield foods, such as sliced meats, fast foods, snack foods, cheeses,

SHAKE THE SALT HABIT

- Use the food guide to check the sodium content of the foods you eat each day to get some idea of how much salt you may be eating. Make adjustments if necessary.
- Read food labels more often to check the amount of sodium in servings.
- Cut back on fast food and other low-response cost, low-yield foods known to be high in sodium.
- Use salt sparingly – at the table and in cooking.
- Steer clear of salty foods, such as sliced meats (unless they are the low-sodium variety), pickled foods, salted nuts, crisps, and snack foods.
- Choose low-sodium foods more often, such as low-sodium vegetable juice, crackers, cheeses, pickles, and soups.
- Select no-salt or low-sodium condiments such as ketchup, mayonnaise, chilli sauce, mustard, and soy sauce.
- Eat more fresh fruits and vegetables (which are low in sodium).
- Flavour your foods with salt-free herbs, spices, lemon juice, and extracts.
- Use salt substitutes.

baked goods, and cereals, are loaded with sodium. So are canned foods and pickled cucumbers. Carbonated soft drinks also contain sodium.

Salty foods also tend to be high in fat – a combination that is addictive in its taste appeal and compels you to devour greasy foods like crisps in ever-increasing amounts. (Sodium comes in many forms; see the table on page 148 for examples.)

If you are overweight, you absolutely must watch your sodium intake. In a twenty-year study of nearly 10, 000 people, for each additional 1¼ teaspoons of salt eaten by people who

LABEL LINGO – SODIUM

If you monitor sodium, learn how to interpret food labels to understand labelling that refers to sodium content. For example:

Low salt/sodium: No more than 40 milligrams per serving.

No added salt: No salt or sodium has been added to the food or any of its ingredients.

Reduced sodium: The food contains 25 per cent less sodium than usual.

Salt free: No more than 5 milligrams per serving.

were overweight, the risk of dying from heart disease increased 61 per cent and the risk of dying from a stroke increased 89 per cent. Among people who were of normal weight, extra salt did not confer an extra risk. The reason for this effect is most likely because a high-sodium diet can promote high blood pressure – an established risk factor for heart disease – or aggravate it, particularly in people who are salt sensitive (meaning that even a small amount of salt can trigger a rise in blood pressure).

Whether you are salt sensitive or not, regardless of your blood pressure, cutting back on salt is still a wise move. Most of us eat too much salt anyway, when in reality we require a minimum of 500 milligrams (about a tenth of a teaspoon) and no more than 2,400 milligrams a day (that's about a teaspoon). Your preference for salt may weaken the less you use it in your diet, so start reducing your sodium by controlling the salt-cellar and choosing a greater variety of low-sodium foods. I've listed tips for restricting salt in your diet in the box on page 144.

Abbreviations and Symbols

As you begin to look up the foods in which you're interested, keep in mind the following abbreviations:

carb	carbohydrate
chol	cholesterol
dia	diameter
fl. oz.	fluid ounce
g	gram
mg	milligram
oz.	ounce
pkt	packet
prep	prepared according to recipe or package directions
prot	protein
sat	saturated
serving	serving size identified on a food label
t	trace
tbsp.	tablespoon
tsp.	teaspoon
w/	with
w/o	without
na	information not available
0	zero (no nutrient value)

(Note: A designation of 'na' does not mean an absence of a particular nutrient, only that analysis of that food for that nutrient is lacking.)

All of the nutrient data in *The Ultimate Weight Solution Food Guide* is based on information from the United States government, from producers of brand-name foods, and from fast-food restaurant chains. Also consulted were scientific journal articles that analysed nutrient content of various foods.

We all do better when we know that there are certain consequences to what we choose. This is specific information that will help you better evaluate your foods and stop sabotaging your health and your weight. Choose better foods this time, and you will choose a different outcome – weight loss freedom! Use this guide as part of your accountability system. I suggest that you keep it close by, taking it wherever you go – from the supermarket to restaurants. It will help you make common-sense food choices that let you achieve and remain at your get-real weight.

HIDDEN SOURCES OF SUGARS AND SODIUM IN FOODS

Sugars
Beet sugar
Brown sugar
Cane sugar
Corn sweetener
Corn syrup
Dextrin
Dextrose
Fructose
Galactose
Glucose
High fructose corn syrup
Honey
Lactose
Levulose
Maltodextrin
Maltose
Mannitol*
Maple syrup
Molasses
Raw sugar
Sorbitol*
Sucrose
White grape juice
Xylitol*

Sodium
Baking powder
Baking soda (sodium bicarbonate)
Brine (salt and water)
Disodium inosinate
Disodium phosphate
Monosodium glutamate (MSG)
Salt (sodium chloride)
Sodium alginate
Sodium ascorbate
Sodium benzoate
Sodium caseinate
Sodium citrate
Sodium hydroxide
Sodium nitrate
Sodium proprionate
Sodium saccharin

* These are sugar alcohols, produced from fruit or dextrose. All three contain the same number of calories as sugar. One of the main differences is that they are absorbed more slowly in the body than sugar is, and therefore are believed to be better for people with diabetes, who must maintain good blood sugar control. Sugar alcohols do not lead to tooth decay, unlike other sugars.

The Ultimate
Weight Solution
Food Guide

HIGH-RESPONSE COST, HIGH-YIELD FOODS: BEEF

Food	Serving	Calories	Prot (g)	Carb (g)
Minced, Lean				
Mince, 85% lean, pan-browned	3 oz.	218	24	0
Mince, 85% lean, grilled	3 oz.	197	21	0
Mince, 90% lean, pan-browned	3 oz.	196	24	0
Mince, 90% lean, grilled	3 oz.	173	21	0
Mince, 95% lean, pan-browned	3 oz.	164	25	0
Mince, 95% lean, grilled	3 oz.	139	22	0
Beef, Lean Cuts				
Bottom round, lean only, trimmed to 0" fat, all grades, roasted	4 oz.	207	33	0
Bottom round, lean only, trimmed to 0" fat, choice, roasted	4 oz.	219	33	0

Fat/Sat Fat (g)	Chol (mg)	Fibre (g)	Sugars (g)	Sodium (mg)
13/5	77	0	0	76
12/5	73	0	0	67
10/4	76	0	0	74
9/4	70	0	0	64
6/3	76	0	0	72
5/2	65	0	0	60

Fat/Sat Fat (g)	Chol (mg)	Fibre (g)	Sugars (g)	Sodium (mg)
8/2.5	88	0	0	75
9/3	88	0	0	75

Beef (cont.)	Serving	Calories	Prot (g)	Carb (g)
Bottom round, lean only, trimmed to 0" fat, select, roasted	4 oz.	194	33	0
Bottom round, lean only, trimmed to 6 mm/¼" fat, all grades, roasted	4 oz.	214	33	0
Bottom round, lean only, trimmed to 6 mm/¼" fat, choice, roasted	4 oz.	224	33	0
Bottom round, lean only, trimmed to 6 mm/¼" fat, select, roasted	4 oz.	203	33	0
Bottom round, lean and fat, trimmed to 3 mm/⅛" fat, all grades, roasted	4 oz.	260	31	0
Bottom round, lean and fat, trimmed to 3 mm/⅛" fat, select, roasted	4 oz.	248	31	0
Eye of the round, lean only, trimmed to 0" fat, all grades, roasted	4 oz.	188	33	0

Fat/Sat Fat (g)	Chol (mg)	Fibre (g)	Sugars (g)	Sodium (mg)
6/2	88	0	0	75
8/3	88	0	0	75
9/3	88	0	0	75
7/2	88	0	0	75
14/5	90	0	0	73
13/5	90	0	0	73
5/2	78	0	0	70

Beef (cont.)	Serving	Calories	Prot (g)	Carb (g)
Eye of the round, lean only, trimmed to 0" fat, choice, roasted	4 oz.	198	33	0
Eye of the round, lean only, trimmed to 0" fat, select, roasted	4 oz.	176	33	0
Eye of the round, lean only, trimmed to 6 mm/¼" fat, select, roasted	4 oz.	181	33	0
Eye of the round, lean and fat, trimmed to 0" fat, select, roasted	4 oz.	182	33	0
Flank steak, lean only, trimmed to 0" fat, choice, grilled	4 oz.	235	31	0
Flank steak, lean and fat, trimmed to 0" fat, choice, grilled	4 oz.	256	30	0
Porterhouse steak, lean only, trimmed to 0" fat, all grades, grilled	4 oz.	240	30	0

Fat/Sat Fat (g)	Chol (mg)	Fibre (g)	Sugars (g)	Sodium (mg)
6/2	78	0	0	70
4/1	78	0	0	70
5/2	78	0	0	70
5/2	78	0	0	70
11.5/5	76	0	0	94
14/6	77	0	0	92
13/4	70	0	0	78

Beef (cont.)	Serving	Calories	Prot (g)	Carb (g)
Porterhouse steak, lean only, trimmed to 0" fat, choice, grilled	4 oz.	254	29	0
Porterhouse steak, lean only, trimmed to 0" fat, select, grilled	4 oz.	220	30	0
Porterhouse steak, lean only, trimmed to 6 mm/¼" fat, choice, grilled	4 oz.	244	30	0
Porterhouse steak, lean only, trimmed to 6 mm/¼" fat, select, grilled	4 oz.	230	31	0
Round, tip round, lean only, trimmed to 0" fat, all grades, roasted	4 oz.	199	33	0
Round, tip round, lean only, trimmed to 0" fat, choice, roasted	4 oz.	204	33	0
Round, tip round, lean only, trimmed to 0" fat, select, roasted	4 oz.	193	32.5	0

Fat/Sat Fat (g)	Chol (mg)	Fibre (g)	Sugars (g)	Sodium (mg)
14.5/5	74	0	0	78
10/4	66	0	0	78
13/4	78	0	0	78
11/4	66	0	0	78
7/2	92	0	0	74
7/2.5	92	0	0	74
6/2	92	0	0	74

Beef (cont.)	Serving	Calories	Prot (g)	Carb (g)
Round, tip round, lean only, trimmed to 6 mm/¼" fat, all grades, roasted	4 oz.	210	32.5	0
Round, tip round, lean only, trimmed to 6 mm/¼" fat, choice, roasted	4 oz.	213	32.5	0
Round, tip round, lean only, trimmed to 6 mm/¼" fat, select, roasted	4 oz.	204	32.5	0
Round, tip round, lean and fat, trimmed to 0" fat all grades, roasted	4 oz.	216	32	0
Round, tip round, lean and fat, trimmed to 0" fat, choice, roasted	4 oz.	227	32	0
Round, tip round, lean and fat, trimmed to 0" fat, select, roasted	4 oz.	211	32	0
Round, tip round, lean and fat, trimmed to 3 mm/⅛" fat, all grades, roasted	4 oz.	248	31	0

Fat/Sat Fat (g)	Chol (mg)	Fibre (g)	Sugars (g)	Sodium (mg)
8/3	92	0	0	74
8/3	92	0	0	74
7/2.5	92	0	0	74
9/3	92	0	0	73
10/4	93	0	0	73
8/3	92	0	0	73
13/5	93	0	0	71

Beef (cont.)	Serving	Calories	Prot (g)	Carb (g)
Round, tip round, lean and fat, trimmed to 3 mm/⅛" fat, choice, roasted	4 oz.	258	31	0
Round, tip round, lean and fat, trimmed to 3 mm/⅛" fat, select, roasted	4 oz.	238	31	0
T-bone steak, lean only, trimmed to 0" fat, all grades, grilled	4 oz.	214	29	0
T-bone steak, lean only, trimmed to 0" fat, choice, grilled	4 oz.	224	29	0
T-bone steak, lean only, trimmed to 0" fat, select, grilled	4 oz.	201	29	0
T-bone steak, lean only, trimmed to 6 mm/¼" fat, all grades, grilled	4 oz.	229	31	0
T-bone steak, lean only, trimmed to 6 mm/¼" fat, choice, grilled	4 oz.	232	30	0

Fat/Sat Fat (g)	Chol (mg)	Fibre (g)	Sugars (g)	Sodium (mg)
14/5	93	0	0	71
12/4	93	0	0	73
10/3.5	62	0	0	80
11/4	63	0	0	80
8/3	61	0	0	80
11/4	65	0	0	85
11/4	67	0	0	87

Beef (cont.)	Serving	Calories	Prot (g)	Carb (g)
T-bone steak, lean only, trimmed to 6 mm/¼" fat, select, grilled	4 oz.	224	31	0
Tenderloin, lean only, trimmed to 0" fat, choice, grilled (filet mignon, beef medallions)	4 oz.	240	32	0
Top round, lean only, trimmed to 0" fat, all grades, braised	4 oz.	226	41	0
Top round, lean and fat, trimmed to 0" fat, choice, braised	4 oz.	245	40	0
Top round, lean only, trimmed to 0" fat, select, braised	4 oz.	215	41	0
Top round, lean and fat, trimmed to 0" fat, select, braised	4 oz.	227	40	0

Fat/Sat Fat (g)	Chol (mg)	Fibre (g)	Sugars (g)	Sodium (mg)
10/4	60	0	0	80
11/4	95	0	0	71
6/2	102	0	0	51
8/3	102	0	0	51
5/1.5	102	0	0	51
6/2	102	0	0	51

Beef (cont.)	Serving	Calories	Prot (g)	Carb (g)
Top round, lean only, trimmed to 6 mm/¼" fat, all grades, grilled	4 oz.	232	41	0
Top round, lean only, trimmed to 6 mm/¼" fat, all grades, grilled	4 oz.	204	36	0
Top round, lean and fat only, trimmed to 3 mm/⅛" fat, select, grilled	4 oz.	222	35	0
Top sirloin, lean only, trimmed to 0" fat, all grades, grilled	4 oz.	216	34	0
Top sirloin, lean only, trimmed to 0" fat, choice, grilled	4 oz.	227	34	0
Top sirloin, lean only, trimmed to 0" fat, select, grilled	4 oz.	204	34	0
Top sirloin, lean only, trimmed to 6 mm/¼" fat, all grades, grilled	4 oz.	221	34	0

Fat/Sat Fat (g)	Chol (mg)	Fibre (g)	Sugars (g)	Sodium (mg)
6/2	102	0	0	51
5.5/2	95	0	0	69
8/3	96	0	0	68
8/3	101	0	0	75
9/3.5	101	0	0	75
6/2.5	101	0	0	75
8/3	101	0	0	75

Beef (cont.)	Serving	Calories	Prot (g)	Carb (g)
Top sirloin, lean only, trimmed to 6 mm/¼" fat, choice, grilled	4 oz.	229	34	0
Top sirloin, lean only, trimmed to choice, 6 mm/¼" fat, select, grilled	4 oz.	211	34	0
Top sirloin, lean and fat, trimmed to 0" fat, all grades, grilled	4 oz.	244	33	0
Top sirloin, lean and fat, trimmed to 0" fat, choice, grilled	4 oz.	260	33	0
Top sirloin, lean and fat, trimmed to 0" fat, select, grilled	4 oz.	221	34	0

Variety Meats,* Lean

Beef heart, simmered	4 oz.	198	33	0
Beef kidneys, simmered	4 oz.	163	29	1
Beef liver, braised	4 oz.	182	28	4

* Although relatively low in fat, organ meats are high in dietary cholesterol.

Fat/Sat Fat (g)	Chol (mg)	Fibre (g)	Sugars (g)	Sodium (mg)
9/3.5	101	0	0	75
7/3	101	0	0	75
11/4.5	101	0	0	74
13/5	101	0	0	73
8.5/3	101	0	0	74
6/2	219	0	0	71
4/1	439	0	0	152
6/2	441	0	0	79

HIGH-RESPONSE COST,
HIGH-YIELD FOODS: BEVERAGES

Food	Serving	Calories	Prot (g)	Carb (g)
Coffee				
Brewed	1 cup	5	t	1
Brewed, decaf	1 cup	5	t	1
Espresso, restaurant prepared	100 grams	9	t	1.5
Instant	1 cup	5	t	1
Instant, decaf	1 cup	4	t	t
Sugar-Free				
Carbonated/mineral water	1 cup	0	0	0
Diet soft drinks	1 can (12 fl. oz.)	0	t	t
Soda water	1 can (12 fl. oz.)	0	0	0
Tap water	1 cup	0	0	0
Beverages/Tea				
Brewed	1 cup	2	0	t
Brewed, decaf	1 cup	2	0	1
Chamomile, brewed	1 cup	2	0	t

Fat/Sat Fat (g)	Chol (mg)	Fibre (g)	Sugars (g)	Sodium (mg)
0/0	0	0	0	5
0/0	0	0	0	5
t/t	0	0	0	14
0/0	0	0	0	7
0/0	0	0	0	0
0/0	0	0	0	2
0/0	0	0	t	21
0/0	0	0	0	75
0	0	0	0	5
0/0	0	0	0	7
0/0	0	0	0	na
0/0	0	0	0	2

Beverages (cont.)	Serving	Calories	Prot (g)	Carb (g)
Herbal, brewed	1 cup	2	0	t
Instant, unsweetened	1 cup	2	0	t
Instant, unsweetened, lemon-flavoured	1 cup	5	0	1
Sugar-free, low-calorie, w/ aspartame	1 cup	3	t	t
Sugar-free, low-calorie, lemon-flavoured w/ saccharin	1 cup	5	0	1

Fat/Sat Fat (g)	Chol (mg)	Fibre (g)	Sugars (g)	Sodium (mg)
0/0	0	0	0	2
0/0	0	0	0	7
0/0	0	0	0	14
0/0	0	0	t	2
0/0	0	0	0	24

HIGH-RESPONSE COST, HIGH-YIELD FOODS: BREADS, BREAD PRODUCTS, AND SAVOURY BISCUITS

Food	Serving	Calories	Prot (g)	Carb (g)
Breads and Bread Products				
Bagel, oat bran	8 cm/3" dia	176	7	37
Bagel, plain, enriched	8 cm/3" dia	190	7	37
Cracked wheat bread	1 slice	65	2	12
Egg bread	1 slice	115	4	19
Mixed grain bread	1 slice	65	3	12
Oat bran bread	1 slice	71	3	12
Oat bran bread, reduced-calorie	1 slice	46	2	10
Oatmeal bread	1 slice	73	2	13
Oatmeal bread, reduced-calorie	1 slice	48	2	10
Pitta bread, wholewheat	10 cm/4" dia	74	3	15
Protein bread	1 slice	47	2	8
Pumpernickel bread	1 slice	65	2	12
Raisin bread	1 slice	71	2	14

Fat/Sat Fat (g)	Chol (mg)	Fibre (g)	Sugars (g)	Sodium (mg)
l/t	0	2.5	na	350
l/t	0	2	na	368
l/t	0	1.4	na	135
2/t	20	1	na	197
l/t	0	2	na	127
l/t	0	1	na	122
l/t	0	3	na	81
l/t	0	1	na	162
t/t	0	na	na	89
l/t	0	2	na	149
t/t	0	1	na	104
t/t	0	2	na	174
l/t	0	1	na	101

Breads (cont.)	Serving	Calories	Prot (g)	Carb (g)
Rice bran bread	1 slice	66	2	12
Rye bread	1 slice	83	3	15
Rye bread, reduced calorie	1 slice	47	2	9
Tortilla, corn (not fried)	1 medium (15 cm/6" dia)	42	1	9
Tortilla, wholemeal	1 medium (18 cm/7" dia)	84	3	23
Wheatberry bread	1 slice	65	2	12
Wheat bran bread	1 slice	89	3	17
Wheat bread, reduced-calorie	1 slice	46	2	10
Wheatgerm bread	1 slice	73	3	13.5
Wholemeal bread	1 slice	69	3	13

Muffins

	Serving	Calories	Prot (g)	Carb (g)
Muffin, wheat	1 muffin	127	5	26
Muffin, wholemeal	1 muffin	134	6	27
Muffin, wholemeal, toasted	1 muffin	135	6	27
Oat bran American-style muffin	1 small	178	5	32

Fat/Sat Fat (g)	Chol (mg)	Fibre (g)	Sugars (g)	Sodium (mg)
1/t	0	1	na	119
1/2	0	2	na	211
t/t	0	3	na	93
.5/t	na	1	na	31
.5/t	na	2	na	196
1/t	0	1	na	132
1/t	0	1.5	na	175
t/t	0	3	na	118
t/t	0	t	na	155
1/t	0	2	na	148

Fat/Sat Fat (g)	Chol (mg)	Fibre (g)	Sugars (g)	Sodium (mg)
1/t	0	3	na	218
1/t	0	4	na	420
1/t	0	5	na	422
5/1	0	3	na	259

Breads (cont.)	Serving	Calories	Prot (g)	Carb (g)
Oat bran American-style muffin	1 mini	46	1	8
Oat bran, American-style muffin prepared from recipe, made w/semi-skimmed milk	1 muffin	169	4	24

Savoury Crackers

Crispbread, rye	2 crackers	74	2	16
Crispbread, rye, (triple cracker)	1 cracker	92	2	21
Flatbread	3 crackers	63	1	14
Matzo, wholewheat	1 matzo	98	4	22
Melba toast, rye	4 toasts	76	2	15
Melba toast, wheat	4 toasts	76	3	15
Rye wafers, plain	2 wafers	74	2	18
Rye wafers, seasoned, large (triple)	1 wafer	84	2	16
Wholemeal crackers	4 crackers	72	1	10
Wholemeal crackers, low salt	4 crackers	72	1	11

Fat/Sat Fat (g)	Chol (mg)	Fibre (g)	Sugars (g)	Sodium (mg)
l/t	0	1	na	67
7/l	22	2	na	266

Fat/Sat Fat (g)	Chol (mg)	Fibre (g)	Sugars (g)	Sodium (mg)
t/t	0	3	na	52
t/t	0	4	na	66
t/t	0	3	na	45
t/t	0	3	na	1
l/t	0	2	na	180
t/t	0	2	na	168
t/t	0	5	na	174
2/t	0	5	na	195
3/t	0	2	na	104
3/t	0	2	na	40

HIGH-RESPONSE COST, HIGH-YIELD FOODS: CEREALS

Food	Serving	Calories	Prot (g)	Carb (g)
Cereals*				
All Bran	½ cup	108	5	19
Bran Flakes	¾ cup	99	3	21
Fruit 'n Fibre	½ cup	106	3	22
Grape Nuts	½ cup	208	6	47
Oats, instant, plain	½ cup	69	3	12
Oats, old-fashioned, w/o salt	⅔ cup	150	5	27
Oat Bran	½ cup	146	7	25
Rice Krispies	½ cup	115	2	28
Shredded Wheat	1 biscuit	73	2.5	16
Shredded Wheat Bitesize	1 cup	167	5	41
Special K	1 cup	117	7	22
Sugar Puffs	½ cup	114	2	28
Sultana Bran	1 cup	188	5	45
Weetabix	1 biscuit	70	2.2	15

* Some of these cereals may contain added sugar; however, many are high in beneficial fibre.

Fat/Sat Fat (g)	Chol (mg)	Fibre (g)	Sugars (g)	Sodium (mg)
1.4/t	0	10	8	340
0.6/t	0	4	7	240
4.5/0.8	0	2	7	180
1/t	0	5	7	354
1/t	0	2	na	188
3/t	0	4	0	0
3/t	0	6	na	2
0.3/t	0	0.2	3	196
0.5/t	0	2.2	t	2
t/t	0	6	t	3
t/t	0	t	4	224
t/t	0	1	15.5	3
1/t	0	7	19	350
0.4/t	0	2	1	54

HIGH-RESPONSE COST, HIGH-YIELD FOODS: CHEESES

Food	Serving	Calories	Prot (g)	Carb (g)
Reduced Fat				
Cheddar, half-fat	1 oz.	76	9	0
Cottage, plain	4 oz.	101	12	3.1
Cottage, plain, reduced fat	4 oz.	79	13.3	3.3
Mozzarella	1 oz.	72	5.2	0
Mozzarella, part skimmed milk	1 oz.	72	7	1
Ricotta	1 oz.	40	2.6	0.6

Fat/Sat Fat (g)	Chol (mg)	Fibre (g)	Sugars (g)	Sodium (mg)
4.5/2.8	12	0	0	188
3.9/2.3	16	0	3.1	300
1.5/1	5	0	0	300
5.7/3.9	16.2	0	16.2	111
5/3	16	0	0	132
3/2	21.4	0	0	28

HIGH-RESPONSE COST,
HIGH-YIELD FOODS: CONDIMENTS

Food	Serving	Calories	Prot (g)	Carb (g)
Condiments				
Barbecue sauce	2 tbsp	23	t	4
Enchilada sauce	2 tbsp	15	t	2
Horseradish	1 tbsp	7	t	2
Hot pepper sauce	¼ tsp	0	t	t
Ketchup	1 tbsp	16	t	4
Ketchup, low sodium	1 tbsp	16	t	4
Mustard (Grey Poupon)	1 tbsp	15	0	0
Mustard, yellow	1 tbsp	10	t	1
Picante sauce	2 tbsp	10	t	2
Salsa	2 tbsp	9	t	2
Soy sauce, low sodium	1 tbsp	9	1	1.5
Spaghetti/marinara sauce	½ cup	71	2	10
Tabasco sauce	1 tsp	1	t	t

Fat/Sat Fat (g)	Chol (mg)	Fibre (g)	Sugars (g)	Sodium (mg)
t	0	t	na	255
t/t	0	.5	t	77
t/t	0	t	na	47
0/0	0	0	na	32
t/t	0	t	na	178
t/t	0	t	na	3
0/0	0	na	na	360
t/t	0	.5	na	168
t/t	0	0	t	252
t/t	0	.5	na	139
t/t	0	t	na	600
3/t	0	2	na	515
t/t	0	0	na	30

Condiments (cont.)	Serving	Calories	Prot (g)	Carb (g)
Tartar sauce, low calorie	1 tbsp	31	t	2
Teriyaki sauce, generic	2 tbsp	30	2	6
Teriyaki sauce (Kikkoman)	2 tbsp	30	2	4
Teriyaki sauce (Nestlé)	2 tbsp	42	t	7
Vinegar	1 tbsp	2	0	t
Worcestershire sauce	1 tsp	0	0	0

Pickles and Olives*

	Serving	Calories	Prot (g)	Carb (g)
Gherkin	1 spear	5	t	1
Gherkin, chopped	½ cup	13	t	3
Gherkin, large (10 cm/4" long)	1 pickle	24	1	6
Gherkin, medium (9 cm/3¾" long)	1 pickle	12	t	3
Gherkin, small	1 pickle	7	t	2

* While generally low in calories, these foods tend to be high in sodium and should probably be avoided if your physician has advised you to follow a sodium-restricted diet.

Fat/Sat Fat (g)	Chol (mg)	Fibre (g)	Sugars (g)	Sodium (mg)
2.5/t	3	na	na	82
0/0	0	0	na	1380
0/0	0	0	4	1220
1/t	0	0	6	319
0/0	0	0	na	0
0	0	0	0	60

t/t	0	t	na	385
t/t	0	1	na	917
t/t	0	2	na	1731
t/t	0	1	na	833
t/t	0	t	na	474

Condiments (cont.)	Serving	Calories	Prot (g)	Carb (g)
Sour pickled cucumber	1 spear	3	t	1
Sour pickled cucumber, chopped	½ cup	36	t	2
Sour pickled cucumber, large (10 cm/4" long)	1 pickle	15	t	3
Sour pickled cucumber, medium (9 cm/3¼" long)	1 pickle	7	t	1
Sour pickled cucumber, small	1 pickle	4	t	1
Sweet pickled cucumber	1 spear	23	t	6
Sweet pickled cucumber, large (8 cm/3" long)	1 pickle	41	t	11
Sweet pickled cucumber, medium (7 cm/2¾" long)	1 pickle	29	t	8
Sweet pickled cucumber, midget (5 cm/2⅛" long)	1 pickle	7	t	2
Sweet pickled cucumber, small (6 cm/2½" long)	1 pickle	18	t	5

Fat/Sat Fat (g)	Chol (mg)	Fibre (g)	Sugars (g)	Sodium (mg)
t/t	0	t	na	362
t/t	0	1	na	936
t/t	0	2	na	1631
t/t	0	1	na	785
t/t	0	t	na	447
t/t	0	t	na	188
t/t	0	t	na	329
t/t	0	t	na	235
t/t	0	t	na	56
t/t	0	t	na	141

Condiments (cont.)	Serving	Calories	Prot (g)	Carb (g)
Olive, green	5 olives	23	0	t
Olives, ripe, canned, large	1 olive	5	t	t
Olives, ripe, canned, small	1 olive	4	t	t

Fat/Sat Fat (g)	Chol (mg)	Fibre (g)	Sugars (g)	Sodium (mg)
2.5/t	0	na	na	na
t/t	0	t	na	38
t/t	0	t	na	28

HIGH-RESPONSE COST, HIGH-YIELD FOODS: EGGS

Food	Serving	Calories	Prot (g)	Carb (g)
Eggs				
Egg white	2 large	33	7	t
Egg white, dried powder	1 tbsp	53	12	1
Egg, whole, fresh	1 extra large	86	7	1
Egg, whole, fresh	1 jumbo	97	8	1
Egg, whole, fresh	1 large	75	6	1
Egg, whole, fresh	1 medium	66	5.5	.5
Egg, whole, fresh	1 small	55	5	t
Egg, whole, hard-boiled	1 large	78	6	t
Egg, whole, poached	1 large	75	6	t

Fat/Sat Fat (g)	Chol (mg)	Fibre (g)	Sugars (g)	Sodium (mg)
0/0	0	0	0	108
t/0	0	0	0	173
6/2	246	0	0	73
6.5/2	276	0	0	82
5/1.5	213	0	0	63
4/1	187	0	0	55
4/1	157	0	0	47
5/2	212	0	0	62
5/2	212	0	0	140

HIGH-RESPONSE COST, HIGH-YIELD FOODS: FAST FOODS, ALLOWABLE

Food	Serving	Calories	Prot (g)	Carb (g)
Fast Foods/Salads*				
McDonalds:				
Caesar Salad, w/o chicken	I serving	90	7	7
Grilled Chicken Caesar Salad	I serving	210	26	11
Subway (6 grams of fat or less):				
Ham	I serving	110	11	11
Roast Beef	I serving	120	12	10
Roasted Chicken Breast	I serving	140	16	12
Subway Club	I serving	150	17	12
Turkey Breast	I serving	100	11	11
Turkey Breast & Ham	I serving	120	13	11
Veggie Delite	I serving	50	2	9

* Dressing not included

Fat/Sat Fat (g)	Chol (mg)	Fibre (g)	Sugars (g)	Sodium (mg)
4/3	10	3	3	170
7/3	60	3	3	680

Fat/Sat Fat (g)	Chol (mg)	Fibre (g)	Sugars (g)	Sodium (mg)
3/1	25	3	3	1070
3/1.5	20	3	3	720
3/1	45	3	4	800
3.5/1.5	35	3	4	1110
2/0	20	3	3	820
3/.5	25	3	3	1030
1/0	0	3	2	310

Fast Foods (cont.)	Serving	Calories	Prot (g)	Carb (g)

Fast Foods/Sandwiches/Poultry

Burger King:

BK Veggie Burger, w/o mayo	1 serving	310	15	46

Kentucky Fried Chicken:

Honey BBQ Flavoured Sandwich	1 serving	310	28	37

Fast Foods/Soups

Subway:

Minestrone	1 cup	70	3	11

Fast Foods/Subs

Subway (6 grams of fat or less):

Ham	1 15 cm/6" sub	290	18	46
Roast Beef	1 15 cm/6" sub	290	19	45
Roasted Chicken Breast	1 15 cm/6" sub	320	23	47
Subway Club	1 15 cm/6" sub	320	24	46

Fat/Sat Fat (g)	Chol (mg)	Fibre (g)	Sugars (g)	Sodium (mg)
7/1	0	4	7	890
6/2	125	2	7	560
1/0	15	2	0	1080
5/1.5	25	4	7	1270
5/2	20	4	7	910
5/2	45	5	8	1000
6/2	35	4	7	1300

Fast Foods (cont.)	Serving	Calories	Prot (g)	Carb (g)
Turkey Breast	1 15 cm/6" sub	280	18	46
Turkey Breast & Ham	1 15 cm/6" sub	290	20	46
Veggie Delite	1 15 cm/6" sub	230	9	44

Fat/Sat Fat (g)	Chol (mg)	Fibre (g)	Sugars (g)	Sodium (mg)
4.5/1.5	20	4	6	1010
5/1.5	25	4	7	1220
3/1	0	4	6	510

HIGH-RESPONSE COST, HIGH-YIELD FOODS: FATS, OILS, AND SALAD DRESSINGS

Food	Serving	Calories	Prot (g)	Carb (g)
Mayonnaise				
Mayonnaise, regular	1 tbsp	57	t	4
Mayonnaise, reduced-fat	2 tbsp	86	0.3	2.5
Oils				
Almond oil	1 tbsp	119	0	0
Apricot kernel oil	1 tbsp	119	0	0
Avocado oil	1 tbsp	124	0	0
Butter replacement, w/o fat, powder	1 tsp	6	0	1
Corn oil, salad or cooking	1 tbsp	120	0	0
Flaxseed (linseed) oil	1 tbsp	119	0	0
Grapeseed oil	1 tbsp	120	0	0
Groundnut oil, salad or cooking	1 tbsp	119	0	0
Hazelnut oil	1 tbsp	119	0	0

Fat/Sat Fat (g)	Chol (mg)	Fibre (g)	Sugars (g)	Sodium (mg)
5/1	4	0	na	105
8.4/1.3	6.5	0	1.5	282
14/1	0	0	0	0
14/1	0	0	0	0
14/2	na	0	0	0
0/0	0	0	0	20
14/2	0	0	0	0
14/1	0	0	0	0
14/1	0	0	0	0
14/3	0	0	0	0
14/1	0	0	0	0

Fats & Oils (cont.)	Serving	Calories	Prot (g)	Carb (g)
Olive oil, salad or cooking	1 tbsp	119	0	0
Rapeseed oil	1 tbsp	124	0	0
Sesame oil, salad or cooking	1 tbsp	120	0	0
Safflower oil, salad or cooking	1 tbsp	120	0	0
Safflower oil (over 70% safflower) salad or cooking	1 tbsp	120	0	0
Soyabean oil, salad or cooking	1 tbsp	120	0	0
Sunflower oil (less than 60% linoleic)	1 tbsp	120	0	0
Sunflower oil (more than 60% linoleic)	1 tbsp	120	0	0
Sunflower oil (more than 70% oleic)	1 tbsp	124	0	0
Walnut oil	1 tbsp	120	0	0
Wheatgerm oil	1 tbsp	120	0	0

Salad Dressings

Blue cheese, regular	1 tbsp	76	1	1

Fat/Sat Fat (g)	Chol (mg)	Fibre (g)	Sugars (g)	Sodium (mg)
14/2	0	0	0	0
14/1	0	0	0	0
14/2	0	0	0	0
14/1	0	0	0	0
14/1	0	0	0	0
14/2	0	0	0	0
14/1	0	0	0	0
14/1	0	0	0	0
14/1	0	0	0	0
14/1	0	0	0	0
14/2	0	0	0	0
8/1	3	0	na	5

Fats & Oils (cont.)	Serving	Calories	Prot (g)	Carb (g)
Blue cheese low-fat	2 tbsp	60	0	4
Caesar salad dressing, low calorie	2 tbsp	32	0	6
Coleslaw dressing, reduced fat	2 tbsp	112	0	14
French, regular	1 tbsp	69	t	3
French, diet, low-fat	2 tbsp	43	t	7
Italian, regular	1 tbsp	69	t	2
Italian, diet	2 tbsp	32	t	1
Italian, fat-free (Kraft)	2 tbsp	20	t	4
Italian, zesty (Kraft)	1 tbsp	54	t	1
Ranch, regular (Kraft)	1 tbsp	74	t	t
Ranch, fat-free (Kraft)	2 tbsp	48	t	11
Russian, regular	1 tbsp	74	t	2
Russian, low-calorie	2 tbsp	45	t	9
Sesame seed dressing	1 tbsp	66	t	1

Fat/Sat Fat (g)	Chol (mg)	Fibre (g)	Sugars (g)	Sodium (mg)
4/2	10	0	na	480
2/0	0	0	4	324
6/2	8	0	14	544
7/2	0	0	na	219
2/t	0	0	na	252
7/1	0	0	na	116
3/t	2	0	na	236
t/t	1	t	2	430
6/1	0	t	1	253
8/1	4	0	t	144
t/t	0	t	2	354
8/1	3	3	na	130
1/t	2	t	na	278
7/1	0	t	na	150

Fats & Oils (cont.)	Serving	Calories	Prot (g)	Carb (g)
Thousand Island, regular	1 tbsp	60	t	2
Thousand Island, low-calorie, diet	2 tbsp	48	t	5
Vinaigrette, balsamic	1 tbsp	50	0	2
Vinaigrette, red wine	1 tbsp	45	t	1

Fat/Sat Fat (g)	Chol (mg)	Fibre (g)	Sugars (g)	Sodium (mg)
6/1	4	0	na	112
3/t	5	t	na	300
4.5/1	0	0	2	165
4.5/na	na	na	na	na

HIGH-RESPONSE COST, HIGH-YIELD FOODS: FISH AND SHELLFISH

Food	Serving	Calories	Prot (g)	Carb (g)
Fish				
Arctic char or charr, mixed species, cooked	4 oz.	151	24	0
Bass, freshwater, mixed species, cooked	4 oz.	165	27	0
Bass, striped, cooked	4 oz.	141	26	0
Bluefish, cooked	4 oz.	180	29	0
Butterfish, cooked	4 oz.	212	25	0
Carp, cooked	4 oz.	184	26	0
Catfish or wolf-fish, channel, farmed, cooked	4 oz.	172	21	0
Catfish or wolf-fish, channel, wild, cooked	4 oz.	119	21	0
Caviar, black and red, granular	3 tbsp	121	12	2
Cod, Atlantic, cooked	4 oz.	119	26	0
Cod, Pacific, cooked	4 oz.	119	26	0

Fat/Sat Fat (g)	Chol (mg)	Fibre (g)	Sugars (g)	Sodium (mg)
5/1	120	0	0	84
5/1	99	0	0	102
3/1	117	0	0	100
6/1	86	0	0	87
12/na	94	0	0	129
8/2	95	0	0	71
9/2	73	0	0	91
3/1	82	0	0	57
9/2	282	0	0	720
1/t	62	0	0	88
1/t	53	0	0	103

Fish (cont.)	Serving	Calories	Prot (g)	Carb (g)
Dab, mixed species, cooked	4 oz.	212	34	0
Dolphinfish or dorade, cooked (mahi mahi)	4 oz.	124	27	0
Drum, freshwater, cooked	4 oz.	173	26	0
Flounder, cooked	4 oz.	133	27	0
Grouper, mixed species, cooked	4 oz.	134	28	0
Haddock, cooked	4 oz.	127	27	0
Halibut, Atlantic and Pacific, cooked	4 oz.	159	30	0
Halibut, Greenland, cooked	4 oz.	271	21	0
Herring, Atlantic, cooked	4 oz.	230	26	0
Herring, Atlantic, kippered, large (180 x 60 x 6 mm/ 7 x 2¼ x ¼")	1 fillet	141	16	0
Herring, Atlantic, pickled, (40 x 20 x 13 mm/1¼ x ⅛ x ½")	3 pieces	118	6	4

Fat/Sat Fat (g)	Chol (mg)	Fibre (g)	Sugars (g)	Sodium (mg)
8/na	80	0	0	57
1/t	107	0	0	128
7/2	93	0	0	109
2/t	77	0	0	119
1/t	53	0	0	60
1/t	84	0	0	99
3/t	46	0	0	78
20/4	67	0	0	117
13/3	87	0	0	130
8/2	53	0	0	597
8/1	6	0	0	391

Fish (cont.)	Serving	Calories	Prot (g)	Carb (g)
Herring, Pacific, cooked	4 oz.	283	24	0
Mackerel, Atlantic, cooked	4 oz.	297	27	0
Mackerel, jack, canned, boneless	4 oz.	177	26	0
Mackerel, king, cooked	4 oz.	152	29	0
Mackerel, Pacific and jack, mixed species, cooked, boneless	4 oz.	228	29	0
Mackerel, Spanish, cooked	4 oz.	179	27	0
Monkfish, cooked	4 oz.	110	21	0
Mullet, grey, cooked	4 oz.	170	28	0
Opah, pumpkin seed, cooked	4 oz.	129	28	0
Orange roughy, cooked	4 oz.	101	21	0
Perch, mixed species, cooked	4 oz.	133	28	0

Fat/Sat Fat (g)	Chol (mg)	Fibre (g)	Sugars (g)	Sodium (mg)
20/5	112	0	0	108
20/5	85	0	0	94
7/2	90	0	0	430
3/1	77	0	0	230
11/3	68	0	0	125
7/2	83	0	0	75
2/na	36	0	0	26
6/2	71	0	0	80
1/t	97	0	0	117
1/t	29	0	0	92
1/t	130	0	0	90

Fish (cont.)	Serving	Calories	Prot (g)	Carb (g)
Pike, northern, cooked	4 oz.	128	28	0
Pike, walleye, cooked	4 oz.	135	28	0
Pollock, walleye, cooked	4 oz.	128	27	0
Pompano or cordonnier, Florida, cooked	4 oz.	239	27	0
Redfish, Atlantic, cooked	4 oz.	137	27	0
Rockfish or catfish, Pacific, mixed species, cooked	4 oz.	137	27	0
Roe, mixed species, cooked	4 oz.	231	32	2
Saithe or coley, Atlantic, cooked	4 oz.	134	28	0
Salmon, Atlantic, farmed, cooked	4 oz.	233	25	0
Salmon, Atlantic, wild, cooked	4 oz.	206	29	0
Salmon, chinook or king, cooked	4 oz.	262	29	0

Fat/Sat Fat (g)	Chol (mg)	Fibre (g)	Sugars (g)	Sodium (mg)
1/t	57	0	0	56
2/t	125	0	0	74
1/t	109	0	0	131
14/5	73	0	0	86
2/t	61	0	0	109
2/1	50	0	0	87
9/2	543	0	0	133
1/t	103	0	0	125
14/3	71	0	0	69
9/1	80	0	0	63
15/4	96	0	0	68

Fish (cont.)	Serving	Calories	Prot (g)	Carb (g)
Salmon, chinook or king, smoked (lox), cooked	4 oz.	133	21	0
Salmon, chum or dog, cooked	4 oz.	175	29	0
Salmon, chum or dog, drained solids, with bone	4 oz.	160	24	0
Salmon, coho or jack, farmed, cooked	4 oz.	202	28	0
Salmon, coho or jack, wild, cooked	4 oz.	158	27	0
Salmon, pink, canned, solids with bone and liquid	4 oz.	158	22	0
Salmon, pink, cooked	4 oz.	169	29	0
Salmon, sockeye or red, canned, drained solids with bone	4 oz.	173	23	0
Salmon, sockeye or red, cooked	4 oz.	245	31	0
Sardines, canned in tomato sauce, drained solids w/ bone	3 pieces	203	19	0

Fat/Sat Fat (g)	Chol (mg)	Fibre (g)	Sugars (g)	Sodium (mg)
5/1	26	0	0	2267
5/1	108	0	0	73
6/2	44	0	0	552
9/2	71	0	0	59
5/1	62	0	0	66
7/2	62	0	0	628
5/1	76	0	0	97
8/2	50	0	0	610
12/2	99	0	0	75
14/4	70	0	0	472

Fish (cont.)	Serving	Calories	Prot (g)	Carb (g)
Sea bass, mixed species, cooked	4 oz.	141	27	0
Shad, American, cooked	4 oz.	286	25	0
Shark	4 oz.	147	24	0
Smelt, rainbow, cooked	4. oz.	141	26	0
Snapper, mixed species, cooked	4 oz.	145	30	0
Spot, cooked	4 oz.	179	27	0
Sturgeon, mixed species, cooked, boneless	4 oz.	153	23	0
Surimi	4 oz.	112	17	8
Swordfish, cooked	4 oz.	176	29	0
Tilefish, cooked	4 oz.	167	28	0
Trout, mixed species, cooked	4 oz.	215	30	0
Trout, rainbow, farmed, cooked	4 oz.	192	28	0
Trout, rainbow, wild, cooked	4 oz.	170	26	0

Fat/Sat Fat (g)	Chol (mg)	Fibre (g)	Sugars (g)	Sodium (mg)
3/1	60	0	0	99
20/na	109	0	0	74
5/1	58	0	0	90
4/1	102	0	0	87
2/t	53	0	0	65
7/2	87	0	0	42
6/1	87	0	0	78
1/t	34	0	0	162
6/2	57	0	0	130
5/1	73	0	0	67
10/2	84	0	0	76
8/2	77	0	0	48
7/2	78	0	0	63

Fish (cont.)	Serving	Calories	Prot (g)	Carb (g)
Tuna, bluefin, fresh, cooked	4 oz.	209	34	0
Tuna, light, canned in water, drained solids	4 oz.	132	29	0
Tuna, white, canned in water, drained solids	4 oz.	145	27	0
Tuna, yellowfin, fresh, cooked	4 oz.	158	34	0
Turbot, cooked	4 oz.	138	23	0
Whitefish, mixed species, cooked	4 oz.	195	28	0
Whiting, mixed species, cooked	4 oz.	131	27	0
Shellfish				
Clams, mixed species, canned, drained solids	4 oz.	168	29	6
Clams, mixed species, cooked	4 oz.	168	29	6
Crab, Alaskan king, cooked	4 oz.	110	22	0

Fat/Sat Fat (g)	Chol (mg)	Fibre (g)	Sugars (g)	Sodium (mg)
7/2	56	0	0	57
1/t	34	0	0	383
3/1	48	0	0	427
1/t	66	0	0	53
4/na	70	0	0	218
9/1	87	0	0	74
2/t	95	0	0	150
2/t	76	0	0	127
2/t	76	0	0	127
2/t	60	0	0	1215

Fish (cont.)	Serving	Calories	Prot (g)	Carb (g)
Crab, Alaskan king, imitation, made from surimi	4 oz.	116	14	12
Crab, blue, cooked	4 oz.	116	23	0
Crab, dungeness, cooked	4 oz.	125	25	1
Crab, queen or snow, cooked	4 oz.	130	27	0
Lobster, Northern, cooked	4 oz.	111	23	1
Lobster, spiny, or crayfish mixed species, cooked	4 oz.	162	30	4
Oyster, Eastern or American, canned, drained	4 oz.	63	7	4
Oyster, Eastern, or American, farmed, cooked, dry heat	4 oz.	90	8	8
Oyster, Eastern or American, wild, cooked, dry heat	4 oz.	82	9	5
Oyster, Eastern or American, wild, cooked, moist heat	4 oz.	155	16	9

Fat/Sat Fat (g)	Chol (mg)	Fibre (g)	Sugars (g)	Sodium (mg)
1/t	23	0	0	953
2/t	113	0	0	316
1/t	86	0	0	428
2/t	80	0	0	783
1/t	82	0	0	431
2/t	102	0	0	257
2/1	51	0	0	103
2/1	43	0	0	185
2/1	56	0	0	277
6/2	119	0	0	478

Fish (cont.)	Serving	Calories	Prot (g)	Carb (g)
Oyster, Pacific or giant, cooked, moist heat	4 oz.	185	21	11
Prawns, mixed species, canned	4 oz.	136	28	1
Prawns, mixed species, cooked, moist heat	4 oz.	112	24	0
Prawns, mixed species, imitation, made from surimi	4 oz.	114	14	10
Scallop, mixed species, imitation, made from surimi	4 oz.	112	14	12

Fat/Sat Fat (g)	Chol (mg)	Fibre (g)	Sugars (g)	Sodium (mg)
5/1	113	0	0	240
2/t	196	0	0	192
1/t	221	0	0	254
2/t	41	0	0	799
t/t	25	0	0	901

HIGH-RESPONSE COST,
HIGH-YIELD FOODS: FRUITS AND FRUIT JUICES

Food	Serving	Calories	Prot (g)	Carb (g)
Fruits				
Apple, dehydrated, sulfured, uncooked	½ cup	104	t	28
Apple, dried, sulfured, uncooked	5 rings	78	t	21
Apple, raw (7 cm/ 2¾" diameter), with skin	1 fruit	81	t	21
Apple, raw (7 cm/ 2¾" diameter), without skin	1 fruit	73	t	19
Apple, raw, with skin, sliced	1 cup	65	t	17
Apple, raw, without skin, sliced	1 cup	63	t	16
Applesauce, unsweetened	½ cup	52	t	14
Apricot, canned in water, without skin	½ cup	25	1	6
Apricot, canned in water with skin	½ cup	33	1	8

Fat/Sat Fat (g)	Chol (mg)	Fibre (g)	Sugars (g)	Sodium (mg)
t/t	0	4	na	37
t/t	0	3	na	28
t/t	0	4	na	0
t/t	0	2	na	0
t/t	0	3	na	0
t/t	0	2	na	0
t/t	0	1.5	na	2
t/t	0	1	na	12.5
t/t	0	2	na	3.5

Fruits (cont.)	Serving	Calories	Prot (g)	Carb (g)
Apricot, dried, sulfured, uncooked	10 halves	84	1	22
Apricot, raw	2	34	1	8
Apricot, raw, sliced	1 cup	79	2	18
Avocado, raw, all varieties	¼ fruit	81	1	4
Banana (18 cm/7" to 20 cm/7⅞" long), raw	1 fruit	109	1	28
Blackberries, frozen, unsweetened, unthawed	1 cup	97	2	24
Blackberries, raw	1 cup	75	1	18
Blueberries, frozen, unsweetened, unthawed	1 cup	79	1	19
Blueberries, raw	1 cup	81	1	20
Cherries, sour, red, frozen, unsweetened, unthawed	1 cup	71	1	17
Cherries, sour, red, raw, without stones	1 cup	78	2	19
Cherries, sour, red, raw, with stones	1 cup	52	1	12.5

Fat/Sat Fat (g)	Chol (mg)	Fibre (g)	Sugars (g)	Sodium (mg)
t/t	0	2.5	na	4
t/t	0	2	na	0
t/t	0	4	na	2
8/1	0	2.5	na	5
1/t	0	3	na	1
1/t	0	7.5	na	2
1/t	0	8	na	0
1/t	0	4	na	2
t/t	0	4	na	9
t/t	0	2.5	na	2
t/t	0	2.5	na	5
t/t	0	1.5	na	3

Fruits (cont.)	Serving	Calories	Prot (g)	Carb (g)
Cherries, sweet, canned in juice, stoned	1 cup	135	2	35
Cherries, sweet, canned in water, stoned	1 cup	114	2	29
Cherries, sweet, raw without stones	1 cup	104	2	24
Cherries, sweet, raw, with stones	1 cup	84	1	19
Cranberries, raw, chopped	1 cup	54	t	14
Cranberries, raw, whole	1 cup	47	t	12
Currants, black, raw	1 cup	71	1.5	17
Currants, red and white, raw	1 cup	63	2	15
Dates, domestic, natural and dry	5 dates	114	1	31
Figs, dried, stewed	½ cup	140	2	36
Figs, dried, uncooked	2 figs	97	1	25
Figs, raw, large (6 cm/2½" dia)	2 figs	95	1	24.5

Fat/Sat Fat (g)	Chol (mg)	Fibre (g)	Sugars (g)	Sodium (mg)
t/t	0	4	na	8
t/t	0	4	na	2
l/t	0	3	na	0
l/t	0	3	na	0
t/t	0	4.5	na	1
t/t	0	4	na	1
t/t	0	na	na	2
t/t	0	5	na	1
t/t	0	3	na	1
l/t	0	7	na	6
t/t	0	5	na	4
t/t	0	4	na	1

Fruits (cont.)	Serving	Calories	Prot (g)	Carb (g)
Fruit cocktail, canned in juice	½ cup	55	t	14
Fruit cocktail, canned in water	½ cup	38	t	10
Grapefruit, pink, raw, red, and white (10 cm/4" dia)	½ fruit	41	1	10
Grapefruit, canned sections in juice	½ cup	46	1	11
Grapefruit, canned sections in water	½ cup	44	1	11
Grapes, European, red or green, Thompson seedless, raw	1 cup	114	1	28
Grapes, canned in water, Thompson seedless	½ cup	49	t	12.5
Guava, common, raw, without refuse	1 fruit	46	1	11
Kiwifruit, fresh, raw, without skin, large	1 fruit	56	1	13.5
Lemon, raw, without peel (6 cm/2⅜" dia)	1 fruit	24	1	8

Fat/Sat Fat (g)	Chol (mg)	Fibre (g)	Sugars (g)	Sodium (mg)
t/t	0	1	na	5
t/t	0	1	na	5
t/t	0	1	na	0
t/t	0	t	na	9
t/t	0	t	na	2
1/t	0	1.5	na	3
t/t	0	1	na	7
t/t	0	5	na	3
t/t	0	3	na	5
t/t	0	2.5	na	2

Fruits (cont.)	Serving	Calories	Prot (g)	Carb (g)
Lemon, raw, with peel (6 cm/2⅜" dia)	1 fruit	22	1	11.5
Lime, raw (5 cm/ 2" dia)	1 fruit	20	t	7
Mango, raw, sliced	1 cup	107	1	28
Melon, cantaloupe, raw, wedge (⅛ of large melon)	1 wedge	36	1	8.5
Melon, honeydew, raw, wedge (⅛ of 15–18 cm/ 6–7" dia melon)	1 wedge	56	1	15
Nectarine, raw (6 cm/2½" dia)	1 fruit	67	1	16
Orange, raw, (7 cm/2⅞" dia)	1 fruit	64	1	16
Papaya, raw, cubes	1 cup	55	1	14
Papaya, raw, small (11 cm/4½" lg x 7 cm/2¾" dia)	1 fruit	59	1	15
Peaches, canned in juice, halves or slices	½ cup	55	1	14

Fat/Sat Fat (g)	Chol (mg)	Fibre (g)	Sugars (g)	Sodium (mg)
t/t	0	5	na	3
t/t	0	2	na	1
t/t	0	3	na	3
t/t	0	1	na	9
t/t	0	1	na	16
t/t	0	2	na	0
t/t	0	3.5	na	1
t/t	0	2.5	na	4
t/t	0	3	na	5
t/t	0	1.5	na	5

Fruits (cont.)	Serving	Calories	Prot (g)	Carb (g)
Peaches, canned in water, halves or slices	½ cup	29	t	7
Peaches, dried, stewed, without added sugar	½ cup	99	1.5	25
Peaches, dried, uncooked, halves	3	93	1	24
Peaches, raw, large (7 cm/2¾" dia)	1 fruit	68	1	17
Peaches, raw, slices	1 cup	73	1	19
Pears, Asian, raw (5 cm/2¼" long x 6 cm/2½" dia)	1 fruit	51	1	13
Pears, canned in juice, halves	½ cup	62	t	16
Pears, canned in water, halves	½ cup	35	t	9.5
Pear, raw, medium (approx. 2½ per pound)	1 fruit	98	1	25
Persimmons, Japanese, raw (6 cm/2½" dia)	1 fruit	118	1	31

Fat/Sat Fat (g)	Chol (mg)	Fibre (g)	Sugars (g)	Sodium (mg)
t/t	0	1.5	na	4
t/t	0	3.5	na	3
t/t	0	3	na	3
t/t	0	3	na	0
t/t	0	3	na	0
t/t	0	4	na	0
t/t	0	2	na	5
t/t	0	2	na	2
l/t	0	4	na	0
t/t	0	6	na	2

Fruits (cont.)	Serving	Calories	Prot (g)	Carb (g)
Pineapple, canned in juice, chunks, crushed, slices	½ cup	75	t	19.5
Pineapple, canned in water, chunks, crushed, slices	½ cup	39	t	10
Pineapple, raw, diced	1 cup	76	1	19
Plantains, cooked, slices	½ cup	89	1	24
Plantains, raw, medium	½ fruit	109	1	28.5
Plum, raw (5 cm/ 2⅛" dia)	2 fruits	72	1	17
Pomegranate, raw (9 cm/3⅜" dia)	1 fruit	105	1.5	26
Prunes, dried, stewed, without added sugar, pitted	½ cup	133	1.5	35
Prunes, dried, uncooked	5 fruits	100	1	26
Raisins, seedless, not packed	¼ cup	109	1	29

Fat/Sat Fat (g)	Chol (mg)	Fibre (g)	Sugars (g)	Sodium (mg)
t/t	0	1	na	1
t/t	0	1	na	1
l/t	0	2	na	2
t/t	0	2	na	4
t/t	0	2	na	4
l/t	0	2	na	0
t/t	0	1	na	5
t/t	0	8	na	2
t/t	0	3	na	2
t/t	0	1.5	na	4

Fruits (cont.)	Serving	Calories	Prot (g)	Carb (g)
Raisins, seedless, 5 oz, miniature box	1 box	42	t	11
Raspberries, raw	1 cup	60	1	14
Rhubarb, frozen, uncooked, diced	1 cup	29	1	7
Rhubarb, raw, diced	1 cup	26	1	5.5
Strawberries, frozen, unsweetened, thawed	1 cup	77	1	20
Strawberries, raw, sliced	1 cup	50	1	12
Sultanas, not packed	¼ cup	109	1	29
Tangerine (mandarin), canned in juice	½ cup	46	1	12
Tangerine, raw, large (6 cm/2½" dia)	1 fruit	43	1	11
Watermelon, raw, diced	1 cup	49	1	11
Watermelon, raw, wedge (¹⁄₁₆ of melon)	1 wedge	92	2	20.5

Fat/Sat Fat (g)	Chol (mg)	Fibre (g)	Sugars (g)	Sodium (mg)
t/t	0	t	na	2
l/t	0	8.4	na	0
t/t	0	2.5	na	3
t/t	0	2	na	5
t/t	0	5	na	4
l/t	0	4	na	2
t/t	0	1.5	na	4
t/t	0	1	na	6
t/t	0	2	na	1
l/t	0	1	na	3
l/t	0	1.5	na	6

Fruits (cont.)	Serving	Calories	Prot (g)	Carb (g)
Fruit Juices/Unsweetened				
Apple juice, bottled	1 cup	117	t	29
Apple juice, from concentrate	1 cup	112	t	28
Cranberry juice, cocktail, low-calorie	1 cup	45	0	11
Grape juice, bottled	1 cup	154	1	38
Grapefruit juice, from concentrate	1 cup	101	1	24
Grapefruit juice, pink, fresh	1 cup	96	1	23
Grapefruit juice, white, fresh	1 cup	96	1	23
Lemon juice, bottled	1 tbsp	3	0	1
Lemon juice, raw	Yield from 1 lemon	12	0	4
Lime juice, raw	Yield from 1 lime	10	0	3
Orange juice, from concentrate	1 cup	110	2	25
Orange juice, fresh	1 cup	112	2	27

Fat/Sat Fat (g)	Chol (mg)	Fibre (g)	Sugars (g)	Sodium (mg)
t/t	0	t	na	7
t/t	0	t	na	17
0/0	0	0	na	7
t/t	0	t	na	8
t/t	0	t	na	2
t/t	0	na	na	2
t/t	0	t	na	2
0/0	0	0	0	3
0/0	0	0	1	0
0/0	0	0	1	0
t/t	0	t	na	2
t/t	0	t	na	2

Fruits (cont.)	Serving	Calories	Prot (g)	Carb (g)
Pineapple juice, fresh	1 cup	140	1	34
Pineapple juice, from concentrate	1 cup	130	1	32
Prune juice	½ cup	91	1	22
Tangerine juice, fresh	1 cup	106	1	25

Fat/Sat Fat (g)	Chol (mg)	Fibre (g)	Sugars (g)	Sodium (mg)
t/t	0	t	na	3
t/t	0	t	na	3
t/t	0	l	na	5
t/t	0	t	na	2

HIGH-RESPONSE COST, HIGH-YIELD FOODS: GRAINS, GRAIN CAKES, PASTA, AND NOODLES

Food	Serving	Calories	Prot (g)	Carb (g)
Grains				
Amaranth, dry	¼ cup	182	7	32
Barley, pearl, cooked	½ cup	97	2	22
Bulgur or cracked wheat, cooked	½ cup	76	3	17
Couscous, cooked	½ cup	88	3	18
Millet, cooked	½ cup	104	3	20.5
Quinoa, cooked	½ cup	106	6	17
Rice, brown, long-grain, cooked	½ cup	108	2.5	22
Wild rice, cooked	½ cup	83	3	17.5
Pasta and Noodles				
Chinese noodles, chow mein, cooked	½ cup	119	2	13
Corn pasta, cooked	½ cup	88	2	19.5
Egg noodles, enriched, cooked	½ cup	106	4	20

Fat/Sat Fat (g)	Chol (mg)	Fibre (g)	Sugars (g)	Sodium (mg)
3/1	0	7	na	10
t/t	0	3	na	2
t/t	0	4	na	5
t/t	0	1	na	4
1/t	0	1	na	2
1.5/0	0	1.5	na	6
1/t	0	2	na	5
t/t	0	1.5	na	2

Fat/Sat Fat (g)	Chol (mg)	Fibre (g)	Sugars (g)	Sodium (mg)
7/1	0	1	na	99
t/t	0	3	na	0
1/t	26	1	na	6

Grains (cont.)	Serving	Calories	Prot (g)	Carb (g)
Egg noodles, spinach, enriched, cooked	½ cup	106	4	19
Japanese noodles, soba, cooked	½ cup	56	3	12
Japanese noodles, somen, cooked	½ cup	115	3.5	24
Macaroni, elbow, wholewheat, cooked	½ cup	87	4	18.5
Spinach pasta, refrigerated, cooked	½ cup	148	6	28.5
Spinach spaghetti, cooked	½ cup	91	3	18
Wholewheat spaghetti	½ cup	87	4	18.5

Fat/Sat Fat (g)	Chol (mg)	Fibre (g)	Sugars (g)	Sodium (mg)
1/t	26	2	na	10
t/t	0	na	na	34
t/t	0	na	na	142
t/t	0	2	na	2
1/t	38	na	na	7
t/t	0	na	na	10
t/t	0	3	na	2

HIGH-RESPONSE COST, HIGH-YIELD FOODS:
LAMB, VEAL, AND GAME PRODUCTS

Food	Serving	Calories	Prot (g)	Carb (g)
Lamb, Lean Cuts				
Leg, shank half, lean only, trimmed to 6 mm/¼" fat, roasted	4 oz.	204	32	0
Leg, shank half, lean and fat, trimmed to 6 mm/ ¼" fat, roasted	4 oz.	246	30	0
Leg, sirloin half, lean only, trimmed to 6 mm/¼" fat, roasted	4 oz.	231	32	0
Leg, whole (shank and sirloin), lean only, trimmed to 6 mm/¼" fat, roasted	4 oz.	216	32	0
Loin, lean only, trimmed to 6 mm/ ¼" fat, grilled	4 oz.	245	34	0
Loin, lean only, trimmed to 6 mm/ ¼" fat, roasted	4 oz.	229	30	0

Fat/Sat Fat (g)	Chol (mg)	Fibre (g)	Sugars (g)	Sodium (mg)
7.5/3	99	0	0	75
13/5	102	0	0	74
10/4	104	0	0	80
9/3	101	0	0	77
11/4	108	0	0	95
11/4	99	0	0	75

Lamb & Veal (cont.)	Serving	Calories	Prot (g)	Carb (g)
Shoulder/arm, lean only, trimmed to 6 mm/¼" fat, grilled	4 oz.	227	31	0
Shoulder/arm, lean only, trimmed to 6 mm/¼" fat, roasted	4 oz.	218	29	0
Shoulder, whole (arm and shoulder), lean only, trimmed to 6 mm/¼" fat, grilled	4 oz.	238	31	0
Shoulder, whole (arm and shoulder), lean only, trimmed to 6 mm/¼" fat, roasted	4 oz.	231	28	0
Sirloin chop, lean only, grilled	4 oz.	213	31	0
Veal, Lean Cuts				
Breast, whole, lean only, boneless, braised	4 oz.	247	34	0
Cubed for stewing, lean only, braised	4 oz.	213	40	0
Mince, grilled	4 oz.	195	28	0

Fat/Sat Fat (g)	Chol (mg)	Fibre (g)	Sugars (g)	Sodium (mg)
10/4	104	0	0	93
10/4	97	0	0	76
12/4	105	0	0	94
12/5	99	0	0	77
9/3.5	96	0	0	75

Fat/Sat Fat (g)	Chol (mg)	Fibre (g)	Sugars (g)	Sodium (mg)
11/4	131	0	0	77
5/1	164	0	0	105
9/3	117	0	0	94

Lamb & Veal (cont.)	Serving	Calories	Prot (g)	Carb (g)
Leg, top round, lean only, braised	4 oz.	230	42	0
Leg, top round, lean only, pan-fried	4 oz.	207	37.5	0
Leg, top round, lean only, roasted	4 oz.	170	32	0
Loin, braised	4 oz.	156	23	0
Rib, braised	4 oz.	247	39	0
Rib, roasted	4 oz.	201	29	0
Shank, lean only, braised	4 oz.	201	36.5	0
Shoulder, arm, braised	4 oz.	228	40	0
Shoulder, arm, lean only roasted	4 oz.	186	30	0
Shoulder, blade, lean only, braised	4 oz.	224	37	0
Shoulder, blade, lean only, roasted	4 oz.	194	29	0
Shoulder, whole (arm and shoulder), lean only, braised	4 oz.	226	38	0

Fat/Sat Fat (g)	Chol (mg)	Fibre (g)	Sugars (g)	Sodium (mg)
6/2	153	0	0	76
5/1.5	121	0	0	87
4/1	117	0	0	77
6/2	86	0	0	58
9/3	163	0	0	112
8/2	130	0	0	110
5/1	143	0	0	107
6/2	176	0	0	102
7/3	124	0	0	103
7/2	179	0	0	114
8/3	135	0	0	116
7/2	147	0	0	110

Lamb & Veal (cont.)	Serving	Calories	Prot (g)	Carb (g)
Shoulder, whole (arm and shoulder), lean only, roasted	4 oz.	193	29	0
Sirloin, lean only, braised	4 oz.	231	38.5	0
Sirloin, lean only, roasted	4 oz.	190	30	0

Variety Meats, Lean

Veal liver, braised	4 oz.	187	24.5	3
Veal spleen, braised	4 oz.	146	27	0

Game Meats, Lean

Rabbit, domesticated, various cuts, roasted	4 oz.	223	33	0
Rabbit, domesticated, various cuts, stewed	4 oz.	233	34	0
Rabbit, wild, various cuts, stewed	4 oz.	196	37	0
Venison, minced, pan-grilled	4 oz.	211	30	0
Venison, loin, lean only, grilled	4 oz.	170	34	0

Fat/Sat Fat (g)	Chol (mg)	Fibre (g)	Sugars (g)	Sodium (mg)
7.5/3	129	0	0	110
7/2	128	0	0	92
7/3	118	0	0	96

| 8/3 | 636 | 0 | 0 | 60 |
| 3/1 | 507 | 0 | 0 | 66 |

9/3	93	0	0	53
9.5/3	97	0	0	42
4/1	139	0	0	51
9/4.5	111	0	0	88
3/1	89	0	0	64

Lamb & Veal (cont.)	Serving	Calories	Prot (g)	Carb (g)
Venison, roasted	4 oz.	179	34	0
Venison, shoulder roast, lean only, braised	4 oz.	216	41	0
Venison, tenderloin, lean only, grilled	4 oz.	168	34	0
Venison, top round, lean only, grilled	4 oz.	172	35.5	0

Fat/Sat Fat (g)	Chol (mg)	Fibre (g)	Sugars (g)	Sodium (mg)
4/1	127	0	0	61
4/2	128	0	0	59
3/1	99	0	0	64
2/1	96	0	0	51

HIGH-RESPONSE COST, HIGH-YIELD FOODS: MILK, MILK PRODUCTS, AND YOGURT

Food	Serving	Calories	Prot (g)	Carb (g)
Milk and Milk Products				
Buttermilk, low-fat	1 cup	98	8	12
Cocoa, sugar-free mix, mixed with water	1 packet	54	2	11
Dry milk, non-fat, instant	⅓ cup	82	8	12
Evaporated milk, canned, non-fat	½ cup	100	10	15
Semi-skimmed milk	1 cup	115	9	12
Skimmed milk	1 cup	80	9	11
Whole milk	1 cup	165	8	11
Yogurt				
Frozen yogurt, non-fat, w/ low-calorie sweetener	½ cup	100	4	18
Light yogurt (Yoplait)	6 oz.	100	5	19
Non-fat, no-sugar yogurt, vanilla, lemon, maple, or coffee flavour	1 cup	105	10	18

Fat/Sat Fat (g)	Chol (mg)	Fibre (g)	Sugars (g)	Sodium (mg)
2/1	10	0	na	257
t/t	na	1	na	173
t/t	4	0	na	125
t/t	5	0	na	147
4.5/2.5	15	0	12	108
0.7/0.2	9	0	11	110
9.5/6.5	35	0	11	108

Fat/Sat Fat (g)	Chol (mg)	Fibre (g)	Sugars (g)	Sodium (mg)
1/t	3	2	na	75
0/0	t	0	14	85
t/t	5	0	na	144

Milk Products (cont.)	Serving	Calories	Prot (g)	Carb (g)
Plain or sugar-free fruit-flavoured yogurt, low-fat	1 cup	143	12	16
Plain yogurt, skimmed milk	1 cup	127	13	17

Fat/Sat Fat (g)	Chol (mg)	Fibre (g)	Sugars (g)	Sodium (mg)
4/2	14	0	na	159
t/t	5	0	na	175

HIGH-RESPONSE COST,
HIGH-YIELD FOODS: NUTS AND SEEDS

Food	Serving	Calories	Prot (g)	Carb (g)
Nuts and Seeds				
Almonds, dry roasted, w/ salt	1 tbsp	51	2	2
Almonds, dry roasted, w/o salt	1 tbsp	51	2	2
Brazil nuts, dried	1 tbsp	57	1	1
Cashews, dry roasted, w/ salt	1 tbsp	49	1	3
Cashews, dry roasted, w/o salt	1 tbsp	49	1	3
Hazelnuts	1 tbsp	53	1	1
Macadamia nuts, dry roasted, w/ salt	1 tbsp	60	1	1
Macadamia nuts, dry roasted, w/o salt	1 tbsp	60	1	1
Mixed nuts, dry roasted, w/ salt	1 tbsp	51	1	2
Mixed nuts, dry roasted, w/o salt	1 tbsp	51	1	2

Fat/Sat Fat (g)	Chol (mg)	Fibre (g)	Sugars (g)	Sodium (mg)
5/t	0	1	t	29
5/t	0	1	t	0
6/1	0	.5	na	0
4/1	0	t	na	55
4/1	0	t	na	1
5/t	0	1	t	0
6/1	0	1	t	22
6/1	0	1	t	0
4/1	0	1	na	57
4/1	0	1	na	1

Nuts & Seeds (cont.)	Serving	Calories	Prot (g)	Carb (g)
Peanuts, all types, dry roasted, w/ salt*	10 peanuts	59	2	2
Peanuts, all types, dry roasted, w/o salt*	10 peanuts	59	2	2
Pecans	1 tbsp	47	1	1
Pistachio nuts, dry roasted, w/ salt	1 tbsp	45	2	2
Pistachio nuts, dry roasted, w/o salt	1 tbsp	45	2	2
Sunflower seeds, dried	1 tbsp	57	2	2
Sunflower seeds, dry roasted, w/ salt	1 tbsp	52	2	2
Sunflower seeds, dry roasted, w/o salt	1 tbsp	52	2	2
Sunflower seeds, toasted, w/ salt	1 tbsp	58	2	2
Walnuts	1 tbsp	41	1	1

*Peanuts are technically pulses but we tend to think of them as nuts.

Fat/Sat Fat (g)	Chol (mg)	Fibre (g)	Sugars (g)	Sodium (mg)
5/1	0	1	na	81
5/1	0	1	na	1
5/t	0	1	t	0
4/t	0	1	1	32
4/t	0	1	1	1
5/.5	0	1	na	0
5/.5	0	1	na	70
5/.5	0	1	na	0
5/.5	0	1	na	57
4/t	0	t	t	0

HIGH-RESPONSE COST,
HIGH-YIELD FOODS: PORK PRODUCTS

Food	Serving	Calories	Prot (g)	Carb (g)
Pork, Lean Cuts				
Centre loin chop, w/ bone, lean only, braised	4 oz. edible portion	229	34	0
Centre loin chop, w/ bone, lean only, grilled	4 oz. edible portion	229	34	0
Sirloin chop, w/ bone, lean only, grilled	4 oz. edible portion	223	31	0
Sirloin chop, boneless, lean only, grilled	4 oz.	219	35	0
Sirloin roast, boneless, lean only, roasted	4 oz.	224	33	0
Tenderloin, lean only, grilled	4 oz.	212	34	0
Tenderloin, lean only, roasted	4 oz.	186	32	0
Tenderloin, lean and fat, grilled	4 oz.	228	34	0

Fat/Sat Fat (g)	Chol (mg)	Fibre (g)	Sugars (g)	Sodium (mg)
9/3	96	0	0	70
9/3	93	0	0	68
10/4	92	0	0	60
8/3	104	0	0	63
9/3	97	0	0	63
7/2.5	107	0	0	74
5.5/2	90	0	0	63
9/3	107	0	0	73

Pork Products (cont.)	Serving	Calories	Prot (g)	Carb (g)
Top loin chop, boneless, lean only, braised	4 oz.	229	33	0
Top loin chop, boneless, lean only, grilled	4 oz.	230	35	0
Variety Meats,* Lean				
Pork heart, braised	1 heart	191	30	.5
Pork kidneys, braised	4 oz.	171	29	0
Pork liver, braised	4 oz.	187	29	4
Pork spleen, braised	4 oz.	169	32	0

* Although relatively low in fat, organ meats are high in dietary cholesterol.

Fat/Sat Fat (g)	Chol (mg)	Fibre (g)	Sugars (g)	Sodium (mg)
10/4	83	0	0	48
9/3	91	0	0	74

Fat/Sat Fat (g)	Chol (mg)	Fibre (g)	Sugars (g)	Sodium (mg)
6.5/2	285	0	0	45
5/2	544	0	0	91
5/1.5	402	0	0	56
4/1	571	0	0	121

HIGH-RESPONSE COST, HIGH-YIELD FOODS: POULTRY PRODUCTS

Food	Serving	Calories	Prot (g)	Carb (g)
Chicken				
Breast, meat only, roasted	4 oz.	186	35	0
Dark meat, roasted	4 oz.	232	31	0
Light meat, roasted	4 oz.	195	35	0
Duck and Goose				
Duck, wild, breast, w/o skin, cooked	4 oz.	140	22	0
Goose, w/o skin, roasted	4 oz.	268	33	0
Variety and Specialty Poultry				
Liver, chicken, cooked	4 oz.	176	28	1
Ostrich, cooked	4 oz.	160	30	0
Pheasant, w/o skin, cooked	4 oz.	152	27	0
Turkey				
Back meat, w/o skin, roasted	4 oz	192	32	0

Fat/Sat Fat (g)	Chol (mg)	Fibre (g)	Sugars (g)	Sodium (mg)
4/1	96	0	0	84
11/3	105	0	0	105
5/1	96	0	0	87
5/2	88	0	0	64
14/4	108	0	0	88
6/0	716	0	1	56
3/0	108	0	0	88
4/0	76	0	0	40
6/2	107	0	0	82

Poultry (cont.)	Serving	Calories	Prot (g)	Carb (g)
Boneless, roasted, light and dark meat	4 oz.	175	24	3
Breast meat, w/o skin, roasted	4 oz.	153	34	0
Dark meat, roasted	4 oz.	183	32	0
Minced turkey	1 burger, 4 oz.	193	22	0
Leg meat, w/o skin, roasted	4 oz.	180	33	0
Light meat, roasted	4 oz.	177	34	0
Neck meat, w/o skin, cooked	4 oz.	203	30	0
Turkey ham	4 oz.	134	18	4
Wing, w/o skin and bone	1 wing	98	19	0

Fat/Sat Fat (g)	Chol (mg)	Fibre (g)	Sugars (g)	Sodium (mg)
7/2	60	0	na	768
1/t	94	0	0	59
5/2	127	0	0	89
11/3	84	0	0	88
4/1	134	0	0	92
4/1	78	0	0	72
8/3	138	0	0	63
5/1	73	0	1	1031
2/1	61	0	0	47

HIGH-RESPONSE COST, HIGH-YIELD FOODS: SLICED MEATS AND SAUSAGE

Food	Serving	Calories	Prot (g)	Carb (g)
Sliced Meats, Lean				
Chicken, smoked	2 oz.	94	10	t
Chicken breast, without skin, oven-roasted	2 slices	33	7	1
Ham, extra lean	2 slices	73	11	t
Turkey breast, lean	4 oz.	155	35	0
Turkey ham	2 slices	64	10	t
Bacon, Lean				
Bacon, meatless	2 rashers	31	1	1
Bacon, turkey	1 serving	35	2	t

Fat/Sat Fat (g)	Chol (mg)	Fibre (g)	Sugars (g)	Sodium (mg)
6/1.5	30	0	na	544
t/t	15	0	t	457
3/1	26	0	na	800
1.7/0.6	74	0	t	90
2/t	38	0	t	632

Fat/Sat Fat (g)	Chol (mg)	Fibre (g)	Sugars (g)	Sodium (mg)
3/t	0	t	na	147
3/1	13	0	t	170

HIGH-RESPONSE COST, HIGH-YIELD FOODS: SOUPS

Food	Serving	Calories	Prot (g)	Carb (g)
Soups				
Beef broth or bouillon, canned, ready-to-serve	1 cup	17	3	t
Beef broth or bouillon, powder, prepared w/ water	1 cup	20	1	2
Beef broth, cube, prepared w/ water	1 cup	7	1	1
Cauliflower, dehydrated, prepared w/ water	1 cup	69	3	11
Chicken broth, canned, prepared w/ water	1 cup	39	5	1
Chicken broth, cube, prepared w/ water	1 cup	12	1	2
Chicken broth or bouillon, dehydrated, prepared w/ water	1 pkt	16	1	1
Chicken noodle, canned, prepared w/ water	1 cup	75	4	9

Fat/Sat Fat (g)	Chol (mg)	Fibre (g)	Sugars (g)	Sodium (mg)
1/t	0	0	na	782
1/t	0	0	na	1362
t/t	0	0	na	1157
2/t	0	na	na	842
1/t	0	0	na	776
t/t	0	na	na	792
1/t	0	0	na	1113
2/1	7	1	na	1106

Soups (cont.)	Serving	Calories	Prot (g)	Carb (g)
Chicken noodle, chunky, ready-to-serve	1 serving	114	8	14
Chicken noodle, dehydrated, prepared w/ water	1 cup	43	2	7
Chicken vegetable, dehydrated, prepared w/ water	1 cup	50	3	8
Clam chowder, Manhattan style, chunky, ready-to-serve	1 cup	134	7	19
Consommé, canned, prepared w/ water	1 cup	29	5	2
Crab soup, ready-to-serve	1 cup	76	5	10
Cream of asparagus, dehydrated, prepared w/ water	1 cup	58	2	9
Cream of celery, dehydrated, prepared w/ water	1 cup	64	3	10
Gazpacho, ready-to-serve	1 cup	46	7	4

Fat/Sat Fat (g)	Chol (mg)	Fibre (g)	Sugars (g)	Sodium (mg)
3/1	24	na	na	875
1/t	8	t	na	433
1/t	3	na	na	808
3/2	14	3	na	1001
0/0	0	0	na	636
2/t	10	1	na	1235
2/t	0	na	na	801
2/t	0	na	na	838
t/t	0	.5	na	739

Soups (cont.)	Serving	Calories	Prot (g)	Carb (g)
Leek soup, dehydrated, prepared w/ water	I cup	71	2	11
Lentil soup, ready-to-serve	I cup	126	8	20
Minestrone, chunky, ready-to-serve	I cup	127	5	21
Minestrone, canned, prepared w/ water	I cup	82	4	11
Minestrone, dehydrated, prepared w/ water	I cup	79	4	12
Mushroom, dehydrated, prepared w/ water	I pkt	74	2	9
Onion, canned, prepared w/ water	I cup	58	4	8
Onion, dehydrated, prepared w/ water	I cup	27	1	5
Pea soup, dehydrated, prepared w/ water	I cup	101	6	17
Split pea, ready-to-serve	I cup	180	10	30

Fat/Sat Fat (g)	Chol (mg)	Fibre (g)	Sugars (g)	Sodium (mg)
2/1	3	3	na	965
1.5/t	0	6	na	443
3/1	5	6	na	864
2.5/t	2	1	na	911
2/1	3	na	na	1026
4/1	0	1	na	782
2/t	0	1	na	1053
t/t	0	1	na	849
1/t	2	2	na	927
2/1	5	5	na	420

Soups (cont.)	Serving	Calories	Prot (g)	Carb (g)
Tomato, canned, prepared w/ water	1 cup	85	2	17
Tomato, dehydrated, prepared w/ water	1 pkt	78	2	15
Tomato vegetable, dehydrated, prepared w/ water	1 pkt	42	1	8
Vegetable, chunky, ready-to-serve	1 cup	122	3.5	19
Vegetable beef, dehydrated, prepared w/ water	1 cup	53	3	8
Vegetable beef, microwaveable, ready-to-serve	1 serving	128	18	10
Vegetarian vegetable, canned, prepared w/ water	1 cup	72	2	12

Fat/Sat Fat (g)	Chol (mg)	Fibre (g)	Sugars (g)	Sodium (mg)
2/t	0	.5	na	695
2/1	0	t	na	708
1/t	0	t	na	856
4/.5	0	1	na	1010
1/.5	0	.5	na	1002
2/1	9	4	na	1098
2/t	0	.5	na	822

HIGH-RESPONSE COST, HIGH-YIELD FOODS: SOYA AND VEGETARIAN FOODS

Food	Serving	Calories	Prot (g)	Carb (g)
Soya Foods				
Black bean burger	1 burger (2.7 oz.)	115	12	15
Frankfurter, meatless	1 link	118	12	2
Soya beans, boiled, w/salt	½ cup	149	14	9
Soya beans, boiled, w/o salt	½ cup	149	14	9
Soya beans, dry roasted	2 tbsp	101	9	7
Soya burger	1 burger	125	13	9
Soya cheese, mozzarella	2 slices (1 oz.)	120	15	2
Soya cheese, Cheddar	2 slices (0.7 oz.)	120	11	1
Soya milk, plain	1 cup	81	7	4
Tempeh	½ cup	160	15	8
Tofu, silken, firm	1 slice	52	6	2
Tofu, silken, soft	1 slice	46	4	2
Vegetable burger	1 burger	138	18	7

Fat/Sat Fat (g)	Chol (mg)	Fibre (g)	Sugars (g)	Sodium (mg)
1/t	1	5	1.5	499
7/1	0	2	t	224
8/2	0	5	na	204
8/2	0	5	na	1
5/1	0	2	na	0
4/1	0	3	1	385
6/na	na	na	na	na
8/na	na	na	na	na
5/t	0	3	na	29
9/2	0	na	na	7
2/t	0	n	1	30
2/t	0	n	1	4
4/1	0	6	na	411

HIGH-RESPONSE COST,
HIGH-YIELD FOODS: SUGAR-FREE FOODS

Food	Serving	Calories	Prot (g)	Carb (g)
Sugar-Free Foods				
Gelatin dessert, sugar-free	½ cup	8	1	1
Gelatin, unflavoured	1 envelope	23	6	0
Jelly/preserves, low or reduced sugar	1 tbsp	24	0	6
Sugar substitute	1 pkt	4	0	1
Sweets, hard, sugar-free	1 sweet	20	0	5
Syrup, sugar-free	2 tbsp	9	0	2

Fat/Sat Fat (g)	Chol (mg)	Fibre (g)	Sugars (g)	Sodium (mg)
0/0	0	0	0	56
0/0	0	0	0	14
0/0	0	0	4.5	0
0/0	0	0	1	0
0/0	0	0	0	0
0/0	0	0	2	27

HIGH-RESPONSE COST, HIGH-YIELD FOODS: VEGETABLES, NON-STARCHY AND STARCHY

Food	Serving	Calories	Prot (g)	Carb (g)
Vegetables/Non-Starchy*				
Alfalfa sprouts, raw	1 cup	10	1	1
Artichoke, hearts, canned in water	4 oz.	42	3	8
Artichoke hearts, boiled, drained, w/ salt	½ cup	42	3	9
Artichoke, whole, globe, boiled, drained w/salt	1 medium	60	4	13
Asparagus, canned, drained	½ cup	23	3	3
Asparagus, fresh, cuts and tips, cooked, w/ salt	½ cup	22	2	4
Asparagus, fresh, cuts and tips, cooked, w/o salt	½ cup	22	2	4
Asparagus, fresh, spears, boiled and drained, w/ salt	6 spears	22	2	4

* These vegetables can be eaten in liberal amounts on the food plans in this book.

Fat/Sat Fat (g)	Chol (mg)	Fibre (g)	Sugars (g)	Sodium (mg)
t/t	0	1	na	2
0/0	0	1	1.5	332
t/t	0	5	na	278
t/t	0	7	na	397
1/t	0	2	na	347
t/t	0	2	na	216
t/t	0	1	na	10
t/t	0	2	na	216

Vegetables (cont.)	Serving	Calories	Prot (g)	Carb (g)
Asparagus, fresh, spears, boiled and drained, w/o salt	6 spears	22	2	4
Asparagus, frozen, cuts and tips, boiled, drained, w/salt	½ cup	25	3	4
Asparagus, frozen, spears, boiled, drained, w/salt	6 spears	25	3	4
Aubergine, cubes, boiled, drained, w/o salt	½ cup	14	t	3
Aubergine, raw, cubes	1 cup	21	1	5
Bamboo shoots, canned, drained slices, w/salt	½ cup	7	1	1
Bamboo shoots, canned, drained slices, w/o salt	½ cup	12	1	2
Bamboo shoots, raw, pieces	1 cup	41	4	8
Beans, green, canned, w/ salt	½ cup	14	1	3

Fat/Sat Fat (g)	Chol (mg)	Fibre (g)	Sugars (g)	Sodium (mg)
t/t	0	1	na	10
t/t	0	1	na	216
t/t	0	1	na	216
t/t	0	1	na	1
t/t	0	2	na	2
t/t	0	1	na	144
t/t	0	1	na	5
t/t	0	3	na	6
t/t	0	1	na	177

Vegetables (cont.)	Serving	Calories	Prot (g)	Carb (g)
Beans, green, canned, w/o salt	½ cup	14	1	3
Beans, green, fresh, boiled, w/ salt	½ cup	22	1	5
Beans, green, fresh, boiled, w/o salt	½ cup	22	1	5
Beans, green, frozen, boiled, w/ salt	½ cup	19	1	4
Beans, green, frozen, boiled, w/o salt	½ cup	19	1	4
Beans, green, raw	1 cup	34	2	8
Beans, yellow, canned, w/o salt	½ cup	14	1	3
Beans, yellow, fresh, boiled, w/ salt	½ cup	22	1	5
Beans, yellow, fresh, boiled, w/o salt	½ cup	22	1	5
Beans, yellow, frozen, boiled, w/ salt	½ cup	19	1	4
Beans, yellow, frozen, boiled, w/o salt	½ cup	19	1	4

Fat/Sat Fat (g)	Chol (mg)	Fibre (g)	Sugars (g)	Sodium (mg)
t/t	0	1	na	1
t/t	0	2	na	149
t/t	0	2	na	2
t/t	0	2	na	165
t/t	0	2	na	6
t/t	0	4	na	7
t/t	0	1	na	1
t/t	0	2	na	149
t/t	0	2	na	2
t/t	0	2	na	165
t/t	0	2	na	6

Vegetables (cont.)	Serving	Calories	Prot (g)	Carb (g)
Beans, yellow, raw	1 cup	34	2	8
Beetroot, raw	1 cup	58	2	13
Beetroot, raw	2 beets	71	3	16
Beetroot, pickled	2 beets	20	0.8	4
Beetroot, whole, fresh, cooked	2 beets	44	2	10
Beetroot greens, boiled, drained, w/salt	½ cup	19	2	4
Beetroot greens, boiled, drained, w/o salt	½ cup	19	2	4
Beetroot greens, raw, chopped	1 cup	7	1	2
Broccoli, Chinese, cooked	½ cup	10	t	2
Broccoli, boiled, drained, w/o salt	1 large stalk (28–30 cm/ 11–12" long)	78	8	14
Broccoli, boiled, drained, w/o salt	1 medium stalk (19–20 cm/ 7½–8" long)	50	5	9

Fat/Sat Fat (g)	Chol (mg)	Fibre (g)	Sugars (g)	Sodium (mg)
t/t	0	4	na	7
t/t	0	4	na	106
t/t	0	5	na	128
t/t	0	1.2	3.9	84
t/t	0	2	na	77
t/t	0	2	na	343
t/t	0	2	na	174
t/t	0	1	na	76
t/t	0	1	na	3
1/t	0	8	na	73
1/t	0	5	na	47

Vegetables (cont.)	Serving	Calories	Prot (g)	Carb (g)
Broccoli, boiled, drained, w/o salt	1 small stalk (13 cm/5" long)	39	4	7
Broccoli, chopped, boiled, drained, w/o salt	½ cup	22	2	4
Broccoli florets, raw	1 cup	20	2	4
Broccoli, frozen, chopped, boiled, drained, w/o salt	½ cup	26	3	5
Broccoli, frozen, spears, boiled, drained, w/o salt	½ cup	26	3	5
Broccoli, raw, chopped	1 cup	25	3	5
Broccoli, raw, spears	2 spears	17	2	3
Broccoli, raw, stalk	1 stalk	42	5	8
Brussels sprouts, boiled, drained, w/o salt	6 sprouts	49	3	11
Brussels sprouts, boiled, drained, w/o salt	½ cup	30	2	7

Fat/Sat Fat (g)	Chol (mg)	Fibre (g)	Sugars (g)	Sodium (mg)
t/t	0	4	na	36
t/t	0	2	na	20
t/t	0	na	na	19
t/t	0	3	na	22
t/t	0	3	na	22
t/t	0	3	na	24
t/t	0	2	na	17
t/t	0	4.5	na	41
t/t	0	3	na	26
t/t	0	2	na	16

Vegetables (cont.)	Serving	Calories	Prot (g)	Carb (g)
Brussels sprouts, frozen, boiled, drained, w/o salt	½ cup	33	3	6
Brussels sprouts, raw	1 cup	38	3	8
Brussels sprouts, raw	6 sprouts	49	4	10
Cabbage, Chinese (pak-choi or bok-choy), shredded, boiled, drained, w/o salt	½ cup	10	1	2
Cabbage, Chinese (pak-choi or bok-choy), shredded, raw	1 cup	9	1	2
Cabbage, Chinese, cooked	½ cup	7	1	1
Cabbage, raw, chopped	1 cup	22	1	5
Cabbage, raw, shredded	1 cup	18	1	4
Cabbage, shredded, boiled, drained, w/o salt	½ cup	17	1	3

Fat/Sat Fat (g)	Chol (mg)	Fibre (g)	Sugars (g)	Sodium (mg)
t/t	0	3	na	18
t/t	0	3	na	22
t/t	0	4	na	29
t/t	0	1	na	29
t/t	0	1	na	46
t/t	0	na	na	6
t/t	0	2	na	16
t/t	0	2	na	13
t/t	0	2	na	6

Vegetables (cont.)	Serving	Calories	Prot (g)	Carb (g)
Cabbage, red, shredded, boiled, drained, w/o salt	½ cup	16	1	3
Cabbage, red, raw, chopped	1 cup	24	1	5
Cabbage, red, raw, shredded	1 cup	19	1	4
Cabbage, Savoy, raw, shredded	1 cup	19	1	4
Cabbage, Savoy, shredded, boiled, drained, w/o salt	½ cup	17	1	4
Carrots, baby, large, raw	6	34	1	7
Carrots, baby, medium, raw	6	23	t	5
Carrots, canned, mashed, w/o salt	½ cup	29	1	6
Carrots, canned, sliced, w/o salt	½ cup	18	t	4
Carrots, raw, chopped	1 cup	55	1	13
Carrots, raw, grated	1 cup	47	1	11

Fat/Sat Fat (g)	Chol (mg)	Fibre (g)	Sugars (g)	Sodium (mg)
t/t	0	1.5	na	6
t/t	0	2	na	10
t/t	0	1	na	8
t/t	0	2	na	20
t/t	0	2	na	17
t/t	0	2	na	31
t/t	0	1	na	21
t/t	0	2	na	48
t/t	0	1	na	31
t/t	0	4	na	45
t/t	0	3	na	39

Vegetables (cont.)	Serving	Calories	Prot (g)	Carb (g)
Carrots, raw, sliced	1 cup	52	1	12
Carrots, sliced, boiled, drained, w/o salt	½ cup	35	1	8
Carrots, frozen, sliced, boiled, w/o salt	½ cup	26	1	6
Cauliflower, raw	1 cup	25	2	5
Cauliflower, raw, florets	6	20	2	4
Cauliflower, boiled, drained, w/o salt	½ cup	14	1	3
Cauliflower, florets, boiled, drained, w/o salt	6 pieces	25	2	4
Cauliflower, frozen, boiled, drained, w/o salt	½ cup	17	1	3
Cauliflower, green, cooked, w/o salt	⅕ head	29	3	6
Cauliflower, green, raw	1 cup	20	2	4
Cauliflower, green, florets	6	47	4	9

Fat/Sat Fat (g)	Chol (mg)	Fibre (g)	Sugars (g)	Sodium (mg)
t/t	0	4	na	43
t/t	0	3	na	51
t/t	0	3	na	43
t/t	0	2.5	na	30
t/t	0	2	na	23
t/t	0	2	na	9
t/t	0	3	na	16
t/t	0	2	na	16
t/t	0	3	na	21
t/t	0	2	na	15
t/t	0	5	na	35

Vegetables (cont.)	Serving	Calories	Prot (g)	Carb (g)
Celery, diced, boiled, drained, w/o salt	½ cup	14	1	3
Celery, diced, raw	1 cup	19	1	4
Celery, strips, raw	1 cup	20	1	5
Chard, Swiss, chopped, boiled, drained, w/o salt	½ cup	18	2	4
Chard, Swiss, raw	1 cup	7	1	1
Chayote, chopped, boiled, drained, w/o salt	½ cup	19	t	4
Chayote, chopped, raw	1 cup	25	1	6
Chicory, raw, chopped	1 cup	9	t	2
Courgettes, frozen, boiled, drained, w/o salt	½ cup	19	1	4
Courgettes, sliced, boiled, drained, w/o salt	½ cup	14	t	4
Courgettes, mashed, boiled, drained, w/o salt	½ cup	19	1	5

Fat/Sat Fat (g)	Chol (mg)	Fibre (g)	Sugars (g)	Sodium (mg)
t/t	0	1	na	68
t/t	0	2	na	104
t/t	0	2	na	108
t/t	0	2	na	157
t/t	0	1	na	77
t/t	0	2	na	1
t/t	0	2	na	3
t/t	0	2	na	11
t/t	0	1	na	2
t/t	0	1	na	3
t/t	0	2	na	4

Vegetables (cont.)	Serving	Calories	Prot (g)	Carb (g)
Courgettes, chopped, raw	1 cup	17	1	4
Cucumber, peeled, raw, chopped	1 cup	16	1	3
Cucumber, peeled, raw, sliced	1 cup	14	1	3
Cucumber, peeled, raw, large (21 cm/8¼" long)	1	34	2	7
Cucumber, peeled, raw, medium	1	24	1	5
Cucumber, peeled, raw, small (16 cm/6⅜" long)	1	19	t	4
Cucumber, with peel, raw, slices	1 cup	14	1	3
Cucumber, with peel, raw, large (21 cm/8¼" long)	1	39	2	8
Dandelion greens, chopped, boiled, drained, w/o salt	½ cup	17	1	3
Dandelion greens, raw, chopped	1 cup	25	1	5

Fat/Sat Fat (g)	Chol (mg)	Fibre (g)	Sugars (g)	Sodium (mg)
t/t	0	1.5	na	4
t/t	0	1	na	3
t/t	0	1	na	2
t/t	0	2	na	6
t/t	0	1	na	4
t/t	0	1	na	3
t/t	0	1	na	2
t/t	0	2	na	6
t/t	0	1.5	na	23
t/t	0	2	na	42

Vegetables (cont.)	Serving	Calories	Prot (g)	Carb (g)
Grape (vine) leaves, raw	1 cup	13	1	2
Jicama, raw, sliced	1 cup	46	1	11
Kale, chopped, boiled, drained, w/o salt	½ cup	18	1	4
Kale, frozen, chopped, boiled, drained, w/o salt	½ cup	20	2	3
Kale, raw, chopped	1 cup	34	2	7
Kale, Scotch, chopped, boiled, drained, w/o salt	½ cup	18	1	4
Kale, Scotch, raw, chopped	1 cup	28	2	6
Kohlrabi, sliced, boiled drained, w/o salt	½ cup	24	1	6
Kohlrabi, raw	1 cup	36	2	8
Leeks (bulb and lower-leaf portion), boiled, drained, w/o salt	1 leek	38	1	9

Fat/Sat Fat (g)	Chol (mg)	Fibre (g)	Sugars (g)	Sodium (mg)
t/t	0	1.5	na	1
t/t	0	6	na	5
t/t	0	1	na	15
t/t	0	1	na	10
t/t	0	1	na	29
t/t	0	1	na	29
t/t	0	1	na	47
t/t	0	1	na	17
t/t	0	5	na	27
t/t	0	1	na	12

Vegetables (cont.)	Serving	Calories	Prot (g)	Carb (g)
Leeks, chopped (bulb and lower-leaf portion), boiled, drained, w/o salt	½ cup	16	t	4
Leeks, chopped, raw (bulb and lower-leaf portion)	1 cup	54	1	13
Leeks, raw (bulb and lower-leaf portion)	1 leek	54	1	13
Lettuce, shredded, raw, butterhead or round types	1 cup	7	1	1
Lettuce, shredded, raw, cos or romaine	1 cup	8	1	1
Lettuce, shredded, raw, iceberg	1 cup	7	1	1
Lettuce, shredded, raw, looseleaf	1 cup	10	1	2
Lettuce, shredded, raw, radicchio	1 cup	9	1	2
Mushrooms, raw, chestnut or marron	6 pieces	18	2	3

Fat/Sat Fat (g)	Chol (mg)	Fibre (g)	Sugars (g)	Sodium (mg)
t/t	0	.5	na	5
t/t	0	2	na	18
t/t	0	2	na	18
t/t	0	1	na	3
t/t	0	1	na	4
t/t	0	1	na	5
t/t	0	1	na	5
t/t	0	t	na	9
t/t	0	.5	1	5

Vegetables (cont.)	Serving	Calories	Prot (g)	Carb (g)
Mushrooms, canned, drained	½ cup	19	1	4
Mushrooms, boiled, drained, w/o salt	½ cup	21	2	4
Mushrooms, boiled, drained, w/o salt	6 pieces	19	2	4
Mushrooms, raw, enoki	6 pieces (large)	10	1	2
Mushrooms, raw, enoki	6 pieces (medium)	6	t	1
Mushrooms, raw, slices or pieces	1 cup	18	2	3
Mushrooms, raw, whole	1 cup	24	3	4
Mushrooms, raw	6 pieces (large)	35	4	6
Mushrooms, raw	6 pieces (medium)	27	3	4
Mushrooms, raw portabella	4 slices	20	3	4
Mushrooms, cooked, pieces, shiitake, w/o salt	½ cup	40	1	10

Fat/Sat Fat (g)	Chol (mg)	Fibre (g)	Sugars (g)	Sodium (mg)
t/t	0	2	na	332
t/t	0	2	na	2
t/t	0	2	na	1
t/t	0	1	na	1
t/t	0	.5	na	1
t/t	0	1	na	3
t/t	0	1	na	4
t/t	0	2	na	6
t/t	0	1	na	4
0/0	0	3	1	10
t/t	0	1.5	na	3

Vegetables (cont.)	Serving	Calories	Prot (g)	Carb (g)
Mushrooms, cooked, whole, shiitake, w/o salt	6 pieces	59	2	15
Mushrooms, dried, shiitake	6 mushrooms	67	2	17
Mushrooms, canned, straw, drained	½ cup	29	3	4
Okra, frozen, boiled, drained, w/o salt	½ cup	26	2	5
Okra, raw	1 cup	33	2	8
Okra, raw	6 pods	24	1	5
Okra, slices, boiled, drained, w/o salt	½ cup	26	1	6
Okra, whole, boiled, drained, w/o salt	6 pods	20	1	5
Onions, boiled, drained, w/o salt	½ cup	46	1	11
Onions, boiled, drained, w/o salt	1 large	56	2	13
Onions, boiled, drained, w/o salt	1 medium	41	1	10
Onions, boiled, drained, w/o salt	1 small	26	1	6

Fat/Sat Fat (g)	Chol (mg)	Fibre (g)	Sugars (g)	Sodium (mg)
t/t	0	2	na	4
t/t	0	3	na	3
t/t	0	2	na	349
t/t	0	3	na	3
t/t	0	3	na	8
t/t	0	2	na	6
t/t	0	2	na	4
t/t	0	2	na	3
t/t	0	1.5	na	3
t/t	0	2	na	4
t/t	0	1	na	3
t/t	0	1	na	2

Vegetables (cont.)	Serving	Calories	Prot (g)	Carb (g)
Onions, canned, chopped	½ cup	21	1	5
Onions, dehydrated flakes	¼ cup	49	1	12
Onions, frozen, chopped, boiled, drained, w/o salt	½ cup	29	1	7
Onions, raw, chopped	1 cup	61	2	14
Onions, raw, sliced	1 cup	44	1	10
Onions, raw, sliced (6 mm/¼" thick)	1 slice	14	t	3
Onions, raw, sliced (3 mm/⅛" thick)	1 slice	5	t	1
Onions, raw, whole	1 large	57	2	13
Onions, raw, whole	1 medium	42	1	9
Onions, raw, whole	1 small	27	1	6
Onions, raw, chopped, spring or salad (tops and bulbs)	1 cup	32	2	7
Onions, raw, whole spring or salad (tops and bulbs)	1 large	8	t	2

Fat/Sat Fat (g)	Chol (mg)	Fibre (g)	Sugars (g)	Sodium (mg)
t/t	0	1	na	416
t/t	0	1	na	3
t/t	0	2	na	13
t/t	0	3	na	5
t/t	0	2	na	3
t/t	0	1	na	1
t/t	0	t	na	0
t/t	0	3	na	5
t/t	0	2	na	3
t/t	0	1	na	2
t/t	0	3	na	16
t/t	0	1	na	4

Vegetables (cont.)	Serving	Calories	Prot (g)	Carb (g)
Onions, raw, whole spring or salad (tops and bulbs)	1 medium	5	t	1
Onions, raw, whole spring or salad (tops and bulbs)	1 small	2	t	t
Palm, hearts, canned	½ cup	20	2	3
Palm, hearts, canned	3 pieces	28	2.5	5
Parsley, freeze-dried	¼ cup	4	t	1
Parsley, raw	1 cup	22	2	4
Parsley, raw	6 sprigs	2	t	t
Parsnips, raw	1 cup	100	2	24
Parsnips, sliced, boiled, drained, w/o salt	½ cup	63	1	15
Peas and carrots, canned, w/o salt	½ cup	48	3	11
Peas and carrots, canned, w/ salt	½ cup	48	3	11
Peas and carrots, frozen, boiled, drained, w/o salt	½ cup	38	2	8

Fat/Sat Fat (g)	Chol (mg)	Fibre (g)	Sugars (g)	Sodium (mg)
t/t	0	t	na	2
t/t	0	t	na	1
t/t	0	2	na	311
t/t	0	2	na	422
t/t	0	.5	na	5
t/t	0	2	na	34
t/t	0	t	na	3
t/t	0	6.5	na	13
t/t	0	3	na	8
t/t	0	4	na	5
t/t	0	3	na	332
t/t	0	2.5	na	54

Vegetables (cont.)	Serving	Calories	Prot (g)	Carb (g)
Peas, sugar snap/ mangetout, fresh, boiled, drained, w/o salt	½ cup	34	3	6
Peas, sugar snap/ mangetout, frozen, boiled, drained, w/o salt	½ cup	42	3	7
Peas, green, canned, w/o salt	½ cup	59	4	11
Peas, green, fresh, boiled, drained, w/o salt	½ cup	67	4	13
Peas, green, frozen, boiled, drained, w/o salt	½ cup	62	4	11
Peas, pigeon, gandules or gungo beans, fresh, boiled, w/o salt	½ cup	102	6	20
Peas and onions, canned	½ cup	31	2	5
Peas and onions, frozen, boiled, drained, w/o salt	½ cup	41	2	8
Peppers, chilli, green, canned	½ cup	15	t	3

Fat/Sat Fat (g)	Chol (mg)	Fibre (g)	Sugars (g)	Sodium (mg)
t/t	0	2	na	3
t/t	0	2.5	na	4
t/t	0	3.5	na	2
t/t	0	4	na	2
t/t	0	4	na	70
t/t	0	6	na	4
t/t	0	1	na	265
t/t	0	2	na	33
t/t	0	1	na	276

Vegetables (cont.)	Serving	Calories	Prot (g)	Carb (g)
Peppers, hot chilli, sun-dried	6 peppers	10	t	2
Peppers, hot chilli, green, chopped, canned, pods	½ cup	14	1	3
Peppers, hot chilli, green, whole, canned	1 pepper	15	1	4
Peppers, hot chilli, green, chopped, raw	1 cup	60	3	14
Peppers, hot chilli, green, whole, raw	1 pepper	18	1	4
Peppers, chilli, red, chopped, canned	½ cup	14	t	3
Peppers, hot chilli, red, whole, canned	1 pepper	15	1	4
Peppers, hot chilli, red, chopped, raw	1 cup	60	3	14
Peppers, hot chilli, red, whole, raw	1 pepper	18	1	4
Peppers, jalapeño, chopped, canned	½ cup	18	1	3
Peppers, jalapeño, sliced, canned	½ cup	14	t	2

Fat/Sat Fat (g)	Chol (mg)	Fibre (g)	Sugars (g)	Sodium (mg)
t/t	0	1	na	3
t/t	0	1	na	798
t/t	0	1	na	856
t/t	0	2	na	11
t/t	0	1	na	3
t/t	0	1	na	798
t/t	0	1	na	856
t/t	0	2	na	11
t/t	0	1	na	3
t/t	0	2	na	1136
t/t	0	1	na	869

Vegetables (cont.)	Serving	Calories	Prot (g)	Carb (g)
Peppers, jalapeño, whole, canned	1 pepper	6	t	1
Peppers, jalapeño, whole, raw	1 pepper	4	t	1
Peppers, sweet, green, strips, boiled, drained, w/o salt	½ cup	19	1	5
Peppers, sweet, green, chopped, boiled, drained, w/o salt	½ cup	19	1	5
Peppers, sweet, green, chopped, raw	1 cup	40	1	10
Peppers, sweet, green, slices, raw	1 cup	25	1	6
Peppers, sweet, green, large, raw	1 pepper	44	1	11
Peppers, sweet, green, medium, raw	1 pepper	32	1	8
Peppers, sweet, green, small, raw	1 pepper	20	1	5
Peppers, sweet, green, rings, raw	6 rings	16	t	4
Peppers, sweet, green, strips, raw	6 strips	4	t	1

Fat/Sat Fat (g)	Chol (mg)	Fibre (g)	Sugars (g)	Sodium (mg)
t/t	0	1	na	368
t/t	0	t	na	0
t/t	0	1	na	1
t/t	0	1	na	1
t/t	0	3	na	3
t/t	0	2	na	2
t/t	0	3	na	3
t/t	0	2	na	2
t/t	0	1	na	1
t/t	0	1	na	1
t/t	0	t	na	0

Vegetables (cont.)	Serving	Calories	Prot (g)	Carb (g)
Peppers, sweet, red, strips, boiled, drained, w/o salt	½ cup	19	1	5
Peppers, sweet, red, chopped, boiled, drained, w/o salt	½ cup	19	1	5
Peppers, sweet, red, chopped, raw	1 cup	40	1	10
Peppers, sweet, red, sliced, raw	1 cup	25	1	6
Peppers, sweet, red, large, raw	1 pepper	44	1	11
Peppers, sweet, red, medium, raw	1 pepper	32	1	8
Peppers, sweet, red, small, raw	1 pepper	20	1	5
Peppers, sweet, yellow, large, raw	1 pepper	50	2	12
Peppers, sweet, yellow, strips, raw	6 strips	8	t	2
Radishes, oriental, sliced, boiled, drained, w/o salt	½ cup	12	t	3
Radishes, oriental, whole, raw	1 radish	61	2	14

Fat/Sat Fat (g)	Chol (mg)	Fibre (g)	Sugars (g)	Sodium (mg)
t/t	0	1	na	1
t/t	0	1	na	1
t/t	0	3	na	3
t/t	0	2	na	2
t/t	0	3	na	3
t/t	0	2	na	2
t/t	0	1.5	na	1
t/t	0	2	na	4
t/t	0	t	na	1
t/t	0	1	na	10
t/t	0	5	na	71

Vegetables (cont.)	Serving	Calories	Prot (g)	Carb (g)
Radishes, slices, raw	1 cup	23	1	4
Radish, large, raw	1 radish	2	t	t
Radish, medium, raw	1 radish	1	t	t
Radishes, daikon or mooli, slices, raw	1 cup	14	1	3
Radishes, daikon or mooli, whole, raw	1 radish	2	t	t
Rhubarb, raw, diced	1 cup	26	1	6
Rocket, raw, chopped	1 cup	6	t	1
Sauerkraut, canned	½ cup	13	1	3
Seaweed, kelp, raw	1 cup	34	1	8
Shallots, chopped, raw	1 tbsp	7	t	2
Spinach, canned, w/o salt	½ cup	22	2	3
Spinach, boiled, drained, w/o salt	½ cup	21	3	3
Spinach, frozen, chopped or leaf, boiled, drained, w/o salt	½ cup	27	3	5

Fat/Sat Fat (g)	Chol (mg)	Fibre (g)	Sugars (g)	Sodium (mg)
t/t	0	2	na	28
t/t	0	t	na	2
t/t	0	t	na	1
t/t	0	1	na	16
t/t	0	t	na	3
t/t	0	2	na	5
t/t	0	t	na	6
t/t	0	2	na	469
t/t	0	1	na	186
t/t	0	na	na	1
t/t	0	3	na	88
t/t	0	2	na	63
t/t	0	3	na	82

Vegetables (cont.)	Serving	Calories	Prot (g)	Carb (g)
Spinach, raw	1 cup	7	1	1
Spring greens, chopped, boiled, drained, w/o salt	½ cup	25	2	5
Spring greens, chopped, frozen, boiled, drained, w/o salt	½ cup	31	3	6
Spring greens, chopped, raw	1 cup	11	1	2
Sprouts, mung, boiled, drained	½ cup	13	1	2.5
Sprouts, mung, raw	1 cup	31	3	6
Squash, spaghetti, boiled or baked, drained, w/o salt	½ cup	21	t	5
Summer squash, all varieties, sliced, boiled, drained, w/o salt	½ cup	18	1	4
Summer squash, all varieties, sliced, raw	1 cup	23	1	5
Summer squash, crookneck and straightneck, diced, canned	½ cup	14	1	3

Fat/Sat Fat (g)	Chol (mg)	Fibre (g)	Sugars (g)	Sodium (mg)
t/t	0	1	na	24
t/t	0	3	na	9
t/t	0	2	na	43
t/t	0	1	na	7
t/0	0	na	na	na
t/0	0	na	na	na
t/t	0	1	na	14
t/t	0	1	na	1
t/t	0	2	na	2
t/t	0	1.5	na	5

Vegetables (cont.)	Serving	Calories	Prot (g)	Carb (g)
Summer squash, crookneck and straightneck, mashed, canned, w/o salt	½ cup	16	1	4
Summer squash, crookneck and straightneck, sliced, canned, w/o salt	½ cup	14	1	3
Summer squash, crookneck and straightneck, sliced, frozen, w/o salt	½ cup	24	1	5
Summer squash, crookneck and straightneck, sliced, raw	1 cup	25	1	5
Swede, cubes, boiled, drained, w/o salt	½ cup	33	1	7
Swede, mashed, boiled, drained, w/o salt	½ cup	47	2	11
Taro shoots or dasheen, slices, cooked, w/o salt	½ cup	10	t	2
Taro shoots or dasheen, slices, raw	1 cup	9	1	2

Fat/Sat Fat (g)	Chol (mg)	Fibre (g)	Sugars (g)	Sodium (mg)
t/t	0	2	na	6
t/t	0	1.5	na	5
t/t	0	1	na	6
t/t	0	2.5	na	3
t/t	0	1.5	na	17
t/t	0	2	na	24
t/t	0	na	na	1
t/t	0	na	na	1

Vegetables (cont.)	Serving	Calories	Prot (g)	Carb (g)
Tomatillos, medium, raw	1 tomatillo	11	t	2
Tomatillos, chopped, raw	1 cup	42	1	8
Tomatoes, crushed, canned	½ cup	39	2	9
Tomatoes, green, chopped, raw	1 cup	43	2	9
Tomatoes, green, slice or wedge, raw	1 piece	5	t	1
Tomatoes, green, whole, raw	1 large tomato	44	2	9
Tomatoes, green, whole, raw	1 medium tomato	30	1	6
Tomatoes, green, whole, raw	1 small tomato	22	1	5
Tomatoes, orange, chopped, raw	1 cup	25	2	5
Tomatoes, orange, raw	1 tomato	18	1	4
Tomatoes, red, canned, stewed	½ cup	36	1	9

Fat/Sat Fat (g)	Chol (mg)	Fibre (g)	Sugars (g)	Sodium (mg)
t/t	0	1	na	0
t/t	0	2.5	na	1
t/t	0	2	na	161
t/t	0	2	na	23
t/t	0	t	na	3
t/t	0	2	na	24
t/t	0	1	na	16
t/t	0	1	na	12
t/t	0	1	na	66
t/t	0	1	na	47
t/t	0	1	na	282

Vegetables (cont.)	Serving	Calories	Prot (g)	Carb (g)
Tomatoes, red, whole, canned, w/o salt	½ cup	23	1	5
Tomatoes, red, whole, canned, w/ salt	½ cup	23	1	5
Tomatoes, red, canned, with green chillies	½ cup	18	1	4
Tomatoes, red, boiled, w/o salt	½ cup	32	1	7
Tomatoes, red, boiled, w/ salt	½ cup	32	1	7
Tomatoes, red, sliced (6 mm/¼" thick)	1 slice	4	t	1
Tomatoes, red (6 mm/¼ of a medium tomato), raw	1 wedge	7	t	1
Tomatoes, red whole, boiled, w/o salt	2 medium tomatoes	66	3	14
Tomatoes, red, whole, raw	1 large tomato	38	2	8
Tomatoes, red, whole, raw	1 medium tomato	26	1	6

Fat/Sat Fat (g)	Chol (mg)	Fibre (g)	Sugars (g)	Sodium (mg)
t/t	0	1	na	12
t/t	0	1	na	178
t/t	0	na	na	483
t/t	0	1	na	13
t/t	0	1	na	296
t/t	0	t	na	2
t/t	0	t	na	3
1/t	0	2.5	na	27
t/t	0	2	na	16
t/t	0	1	na	11

Vegetables (cont.)	Serving	Calories	Prot (g)	Carb (g)
Tomatoes, red, whole, raw	1 small tomato	19	1	4
Tomatoes, red, stewed	½ cup	40	1	7
Tomatoes, cherry, raw	1 cup	31	1	7
Tomatoes, cherry, raw	1 tomato	4	t	1
Tomatoes, red, chopped, raw	1 cup	38	2	8
Tomatoes, plum, raw	1 tomato	13	t	3
Tomatoes, sun-dried	½ cup	70	4	15
Tomatoes, sun-dried	1 piece	5	t	1
Tomatoes, yellow, chopped, raw	1 cup	21	1	4
Tomatoes, yellow, whole, raw	1 tomato	32	2	6
Tomato paste, w/o salt	¼ cup	53	2	12
Tomato paste, w/ salt	¼ cup	53	2	12

Fat/Sat Fat (g)	Chol (mg)	Fibre (g)	Sugars (g)	Sodium (mg)
t/t	0	1	na	8
l/t	0	1	na	230
t/t	0	2	na	13
t/t	0	t	na	2
t/t	0	2	na	16
t/t	0	1	na	6
t/t	0	3	na	566
t/t	0	t	na	42
t/t	0	1	na	32
t/t	0	1.5	na	49
t/t	0	2.5	na	57
t/t	0	2.5	na	517

Vegetables (cont.)	Serving	Calories	Prot (g)	Carb (g)
Tomato purée, w/o salt	½ cup	50	2	12
Tomato purée, w/ salt	½ cup	50	2	12
Tomato sauce, canned	½ cup	37	2	9
Tomato sauce, canned, w/ mushrooms	½ cup	43	2	10
Tomato sauce, canned, w/ onions	½ cup	51	2	12
Tomato sauce, canned, w/ onions, green peppers, and celery	½ cup	51	1	11
Turnips, cubed, boiled, drained, w/o salt	½ cup	16	t	4
Turnips, mashed, boiled, drained, w/o salt	½ cup	24	1	6
Turnips, frozen, boiled, drained, w/o salt	½ cup	18	1	3

Fat/Sat Fat (g)	Chol (mg)	Fibre (g)	Sugars (g)	Sodium (mg)
t/t	0	2.5	na	43
t/t	0	2.5	na	499
t/t	0	2	na	741
t/t	0	2	na	554
t/t	0	2	na	675
t/t	0	2	na	683
t/t	0	2	na	39
t/t	0	2	na	58
t/t	0	2	na	28

Vegetables (cont.)	Serving	Calories	Prot (g)	Carb (g)
Turnip tops and turnips, frozen, boiled, drained, w/o salt	½ cup	15	2	2
Vegetables, mixed, canned	½ cup	38	2	8
Vegetables, mixed, frozen, boiled, drained, w/ salt	½ cup	54	3	12
Vegetables, mixed, frozen, boiled, drained, w/o salt	½ cup	54	3	12
Water chestnuts, Chinese, slices, canned	½ cup	35	1	9
Watercress, chopped, raw	1 cup	4	1	t
Watercress, raw	10 sprigs	3	t	t

Vegetable Juices

	Serving	Calories	Prot (g)	Carb (g)
Carrot juice, canned	1 cup	94	2	22
Tomato juice, w/o salt	1 cup	41	2	10
Tomato juice, w/ salt	1 cup	41	2	10

Fat/Sat Fat (g)	Chol (mg)	Fibre (g)	Sugars (g)	Sodium (mg)
t/t	0	1.5	na	13
t/t	0	2	na	121
t/t	0	4	na	247
t/t	0	4	na	32
t/t	0	2	na	6
t/t	0	t	na	14
t/t	0	t	na	10

Fat/Sat Fat (g)	Chol (mg)	Fibre (g)	Sugars (g)	Sodium (mg)
t/t	0	2	na	68
t/t	0	2	na	24
t/t	0	1	na	877

Vegetables (cont.)	Serving	Calories	Prot (g)	Carb (g)
Vegetable juice cocktail, canned	1 cup	46	1.5	11

Vegetables/Starchy

Acorn squash, cubes, baked, w/o salt	½ cup	57	1	15
Acorn squash, mashed, baked, w/o salt	½ cup	42	1	11

Beans/Pulses

Aduki, boiled, w/ salt	½ cup	147	9	28
Aduki, boiled, w/o salt	½ cup	147	9	28
Black beans, boiled w/ salt	½ cup	114	8	20
Black beans, boiled w/o salt	½ cup	114	8	20
Borlotti beans, boiled, w/ salt	½ cup	120	8	22
Borlotti beans, boiled, w/o salt	½ cup	120	8	22
Borlotti beans, canned	½ cup	108	7	20

Fat/Sat Fat (g)	Chol (mg)	Fibre (g)	Sugars (g)	Sodium (mg)
t/t	0	2	na	653
t/t	0	4.5	na	4
t/t	0	3	na	4
t/t	0	8	na	281
t/t	0	8	na	9
t/t	0	7.5	na	204
t/t	0	7.5	na	1
t/t	0	9	na	210
t/t	0	9	na	1
t/t	0	8	na	432

Vegetables (cont.)	Serving	Calories	Prot (g)	Carb (g)
Broad beans (fava), boiled, w/ salt	½ cup	94	6	17
Broad beans (fava), boiled, w/o salt	½ cup	94	6	17
Broad beans (fava), canned	½ cup	91	7	16
Butter beans, boiled, w/ salt	½ cup	108	7	20
Butter beans, boiled, w/o salt	½ cup	108	7	20
Butter beans, canned	½ cup	95	6	18
Chickpeas boiled, w/ salt	½ cup	134	7	22
Chickpeas boiled, w/o salt	½ cup	134	7	22
Chickpeas, canned	½ cup	143	6	27
Haricot beans, boiled, w/ salt	½ cup	129	8	24
Haricot beans, boiled, w/o salt	½ cup	129	8	24
Haricot, beans, canned	½ cup	148	10	27

Fat/Sat Fat (g)	Chol (mg)	Fibre (g)	Sugars (g)	Sodium (mg)
t/t	0	5	na	205
t/t	0	5	na	4
t/t	0	5	na	580
t/t	0	7	na	224
t/t	0	7	na	2
t/t	0	6	na	405
2/t	0	6	na	199
2/t	0	6	na	6
1/t	0	5	na	359
t/t	0	6	na	216
t/t	0	6	na	1
t/t	0	7	na	587

Vegetables (cont.)	Serving	Calories	Prot (g)	Carb (g)
Kidney beans, boiled, w/ salt	½ cup	112	8	20
Kidney beans, boiled, w/o salt	½ cup	112	8	20
Kidney beans, canned	½ cup	104	7	19
Lentils, boiled, w/o salt	½ cup	115	9	20
Lentils, sprouted, raw	1 cup	82	7	17
Mung beans, boiled, w/ salt	½ cup	106	7	19
Mung beans, boiled, w/o salt	½ cup	106	7	19
Pink beans, boiled, w/ salt	½ cup	126	8	24
Pink beans, boiled, w/o salt	½ cup	126	8	24
Pinto beans, boiled, w/ salt	½ cup	117	7	22
Pinto beans, boiled, w/o salt	½ cup	117	7	22
Pinto beans, canned	½ cup	103	6	18

Fat/Sat Fat (g)	Chol (mg)	Fibre (g)	Sugars (g)	Sodium (mg)
t/t	0	6	na	211
t/t	0	6	na	2
t/t	0	4.5	na	444
t/t	0	8	na	2
t/t	0	na	na	8
t/t	0	8	na	240
t/t	0	8	na	2
t/t	0	4.5	na	201
t/t	0	4.5	na	2
t/t	0	7	na	203
t/t	0	7	na	2
1/t	0	5.5	na	353

Vegetables (cont.)	Serving	Calories	Prot (g)	Carb (g)
Split peas, boiled, w/o salt	½ cup	116	8	21
White beans (small), boiled, w/o salt	½ cup	127	8	23
White beans or cannellini, boiled, w/ salt	½ cup	124	9	23
White beans or cannellini, boiled, w/o salt	½ cup	124	9	23
White beans or cannellini, canned	½ cup	153	10	29

Vegetables/Starchy

Breadfruit, cooked	½ cup	113	1	30
Butternut squash, cubes, baked, w/o salt	½ cup	41	1	11
Butternut squash, frozen, boiled, mashed, w/o salt	½ cup	47	1	12
Corn, air-popped popcorn	2 cups	61	2	12

Fat/Sat Fat (g)	Chol (mg)	Fibre (g)	Sugars (g)	Sodium (mg)
t/t	0	8	na	2
t/t	0	9	na	2
t/t	0	6	na	217
t/t	0	6	na	5
t/t	0	6	na	7

Fat/Sat Fat (g)	Chol (mg)	Fibre (g)	Sugars (g)	Sodium (mg)
t/t	0	5	na	2
t/t	0	na	na	4
t/t	0	na	na	2
t/t	0	2	na	1

Vegetables (cont.)	Serving	Calories	Prot (g)	Carb (g)
Hubbard squash, baked, cubes, w/o salt	½ cup	51	3	11
Hubbard squash, boiled, mashed, w/o salt	½ cup	35	2	8
Potato, baked, jacket, w/ salt	1 medium	161	4	37
Potato, baked, jacket, w/o salt	1 medium	161	4	37
Potato, boiled w/o skin, w/o salt	1 medium	144	3	33
Potatoes, canned, drained	½ cup	54	1	12
Potatoes, micro-waved, jacket, w/ salt	1 medium	156	3	36
Potatoes, red, baked w/ flesh and skin	1 medium	154	4	34
Potatoes, russet, baked w/ flesh and skin	1 medium	168	5	37
Potatoes, white, baked w/ flesh and skin	1 medium	163	4	36

Fat/Sat Fat (g)	Chol (mg)	Fibre (g)	Sugars (g)	Sodium (mg)
t/t	0	na	na	8
t/t	0	3	na	6
t/t	0	4	2	422
t/t	0	4	2	17
t/t	0	3	na	8
t/t	0	2	na	197
t/t	0	2.5	na	379
t/t	0	3	2.5	14
t/t	0	4	na	14
t/t	0	4	3	12

Vegetables (cont.)	Serving	Calories	Prot (g)	Carb (g)
Pumpkin, canned, w/o salt	½ cup	42	1	10
Pumpkin, boiled, mashed, w/o salt	½ cup	25	1	6
Sweetcorn, fresh, white, boiled, drained w/o salt	½ cup	89	3	21
Sweetcorn, white, on the cob	1 ear	59	2	14
Sweetcorn, canned, yellow	½ cup	66	2	15
Sweetcorn, fresh, yellow, boiled, drained, w/o salt	½ cup	88	3	20
Sweetcorn, on the cob, fresh, yellow, boiled, drained, w/o salt	1 ear	83	3	19
Sweetcorn, cut off the cob, frozen, yellow, boiled, drained, w/o salt	½ cup	66	2	16
Sweet potato, baked in skin, w/o salt	½ cup	103	2	24

Fat/Sat Fat (g)	Chol (mg)	Fibre (g)	Sugars (g)	Sodium (mg)
t/t	0	4	na	6
t/t	0	1	na	1
1/t	0	2	na	14
t/t	0	1	na	3
1/t	0	2	na	175
1/t	0	2	na	14
1/t	0	2	na	13
t/t	0	2	na	4
t/t	0	3	na	10

Vegetables (cont.)	Serving	Calories	Prot (g)	Carb (g)
Sweet potato, baked in skin, w/o salt	1 medium	117	2	28
Sweet potatoes, frozen, cubes, baked, w/o salt	½ cup	88	1	21
Winter squash, all varieties, baked, w/o salt	½ cup	40	1	9

Fat/Sat Fat (g)	Chol (mg)	Fibre (g)	Sugars (g)	Sodium (mg)
t/t	0	3	na	11
t/t	0	2	na	7
t/t	0	3	na	1

LOW-RESPONSE COST, LOW-YIELD FOODS: BEEF

Food	Serving	Calories	Prot (g)	Carb (g)
Beef				
Brisket, point half, lean and fat, trimmed to 6 mm/ ¼" fat, all grades, braised	4 oz.	458	25	0
Chuck arm pot roast, lean and fat, trimmed to 13 mm/½" fat, prime, braised	4 oz.	443	30	0
Chuck blade roast, lean and fat, trimmed to 13 mm/½" fat, prime, braised	4 oz.	473	29	0
Corned beef, canned	4 oz.	284	31	0
Corned beef loaf, jellied	4 oz.	171	26	0
Mince, regular	4 oz.	320	28	0
Rib, thick end (ribs 6–9), lean and fat, trimmed to 3 mm/ ⅛" fat, prime, grilled	4 oz.	458	23	0

Fat/Sat Fat (g)	Chol (mg)	Fibre (g)	Sugars (g)	Sodium (mg)
39/15	104	0	na	74
35/14	112	0	na	66
39/16	117	0	na	71
17/7	98	0	na	1141
7/3	53	0	na	1067
22/9	107	0	na	87
40/16	97	0	na	70

Beef (cont.)	Serving	Calories	Prot (g)	Carb (g)
Rib, thick end (ribs 6–9), lean and fat, trimmed to 3 mm/⅛" fat, prime, roasted	4 oz.	445	26	0
Rib, thick end (ribs 6–9), lean and fat, trimmed to 6 mm/ ¼" fat, prime, grilled	4 oz.	468	23	0
Rib, thick end (ribs 6–9), lean and fat, trimmed to 6 mm/ ¼" fat, prime, roasted	4 oz.	456	25.5	0
Rib, thick end (ribs 6–9), lean and fat, trimmed to 13 mm/ ½" fat, prime, grilled	4 oz.	482	22.5	0
Rib, thick end (ribs 6–9), lean and fat, trimmed to 13 mm/ ½" fat, prime, roasted	4 oz.	461	25	0
Rib, thin end (ribs 10–12), lean and fat, trimmed to 3 mm/⅛" fat, all grades, grilled	4 oz.	374	27	0

Fat/Sat Fat (g)	Chol (mg)	Fibre (g)	Sugars (g)	Sodium (mg)
37/15	96	0	na	73
41/17	97	0	na	69
38.5/16	96	0	na	71
43/18	99	0	na	68
39/17	96	0	na	71
28.5/11.5	95	0	na	70

Beef (cont.)	Serving	Calories	Prot (g)	Carb (g)
Rib, thin end (ribs 10–12), lean and fat, trimmed to 3 mm/⅛" fat, all grades, roasted	4 oz.	386	25.5	0
Rib, thin end (ribs 10–12), lean and fat, trimmed to 3 mm/⅛" fat, prime, grilled	4 oz.	401	27	0
Rib, thin end (ribs 10–12), lean and fat, trimmed to 3 mm/⅛" fat, prime, roasted	4 oz.	466	25	0
Rib, thin end (ribs 10–12), lean and fat, trimmed to 6 mm/¼" fat, prime, grilled	4 oz.	409	27	0
Rib, thin end (ribs 10–12), lean and fat, trimmed to 6 mm/¼" fat, prime, roasted	4 oz.	473	25	0
Rib, thin end (ribs 10–12), lean and fat, trimmed to 13 mm/½" fat, prime, grilled	4 oz.	413	27	0

Fat/Sat Fat (g)	Chol (mg)	Fibre (g)	Sugars (g)	Sodium (mg)
31/12	94	0	na	71
32/13	94	0	na	71
40/16	95	0	na	74
32.5/13	95	0	na	70
41/17	95	0	na	74
33/14	95	0	na	70

Beef (cont.)	Serving	Calories	Prot (g)	Carb (g)
Rib, thin end (ribs 10–12), lean and fat, trimmed to 13 mm/½" fat, prime, roasted	4 oz.	476	25	0
Rib, whole (ribs 6–12), lean and fat, trimmed to 6 mm/¼" fat, all grades, grilled	4 oz.	388	25	0
Rib, whole (ribs 6–12), lean and fat, trimmed to 6 mm/¼" fat, all grades, roasted	4 oz.	406	25.5	0
Rib, whole (ribs 6–12), lean and fat, trimmed to 13 mm/½" fat, prime, grilled	4 oz.	462	24	0
Rib, whole (ribs 6–12), lean and fat, trimmed to 13 mm/½" fat, prime, roasted	4 oz.	482	24	0
Sandwich steaks	4 oz.	346	18	0
Short ribs, lean and fat, choice, braised	4 oz.	534	24	0

Fat/Sat Fat (g)	Chol (mg)	Fibre (g)	Sugars (g)	Sodium (mg)
41/17	96	0	na	73
31/13	93	0	na	71
33/13	95	0	na	71
40/17	97	0	na	68
42/18	97	0	na	71
30/13	80	0	0	76
47.5/20	107	0	na	57

LOW-RESPONSE COST, LOW-YIELD FOODS: BEVERAGES

Food	Serving	Calories	Prot (g)	Carb (g)
Alcoholic				
Beer, light	1 can or bottle (12 fl. oz.)	99	1	5
Beer, low-carb (Michelob Ultra)	1 can or bottle (12 fl. oz.)	96	t	2.5
Beer, regular	1 can or bottle (12 fl. oz.)	146	1	13
Cider	1 bottle (12 fl. oz.)	195	0	19
Coffee liqueur, 53 proof	1 jigger (1.5 fl. oz.)	175	t	24
Coffee liqueur, 63 proof	1 jigger (1.5 fl. oz.)	160	t	17
Coffee liqueur w/cream, 34 proof	1 jigger (1.5 fl. oz.)	154	1	10
Crème de menthe, 72 proof	1 jigger (1.5 fl. oz.)	186	0	21
Gin, rum, vodka, whiskey, 80 proof	1 jigger (1.5 fl. oz.)	97	0	0

Fat/Sat Fat (g)	Chol (mg)	Fibre (g)	Sugars (g)	Sodium (mg)
0/0	0	0	na	11
0/0	na	na	na	na
0/0	0	t	na	18
0/0	0	na	na	na
t/t	0	0	na	4
t/t	0	0	na	4
7/4.5	7	0	na	43
t/t	0	0	na	3
0/0	0	0	na	0

Beverages (cont.)	Serving	Calories	Prot (g)	Carb (g)
Gin, rum, vodka, whiskey, 86 proof	1 jigger (1.5 fl. oz.)	105	0	0
Gin, rum, vodka, whiskey, 90 proof	1 jigger (1.5 fl. oz.)	110	0	0
Gin, rum, vodka, whiskey, 94 proof	1 jigger (1.5 fl.oz.)	116	0	0
Gin, rum, vodka, whiskey, 100 proof	1 jigger (1.5 fl. oz.)	124	0	0
Martini	1 fl. oz.	68	0	1
Wine, dessert, dry	1 glass (3.5 fl. oz.)	130	t	4
Wine, dessert, sweet	1 glass (3.5 fl. oz.)	158	t	12
Wine, table, all varieties	1 glass (3.5 fl. oz.)	72	t	1
Wine, table, red	1 glass (3.5 fl. oz.)	74	t	2
Wine, table, rosé	1 glass (3.5 fl. oz.)	73	t	1
Wine, table, white	1 glass (3.5 fl. oz.)	70	t	1

Fat/Sat Fat (g)	Chol (mg)	Fibre (g)	Sugars (g)	Sodium (mg)
0/0	0	0	na	0
0/0	0	0	na	0
0/0	0	0	na	0
0/0	0	0	na	0
0/0	0	0	0	1
0/0	0	0	na	9
0/0	0	0	na	9
0/0	0	0	na	8
0/0	0	0	na	5
0/0	0	0	na	5
0/0	0	0	na	5

Beverages (cont.)	Serving	Calories	Prot (g)	Carb (g)
Coffee and Tea / Flavoured				
Cappuccino-flavoured coffee, powder w/sugar	2 tsp. rounded	62	t	11
Mocha-flavoured coffee, powder	2 tsp. rounded	51	t	8
Lemon-flavoured tea, instant w/sugar	1 cup (8 fl. oz.)	88	t	22
Lemon-flavoured iced tea, ready-to-drink	1 cup (8 fl. oz.)	89	0	20
Soft Drinks				
Cola, w/ caffeine	1 can or bottle (12 fl. oz.)	155	0	40
Cola, w/o caffeine	1 can or bottle (12 fl. oz.)	155	0	40
Cola, w/o caffeine, super-sized, large	1 drink (32 fl. oz.)	413	0	106
Cream soda	1 can or bottle (12 fl. oz.)	189	0	49
Ginger ale	1 can or bottle (12 fl. oz.)	124	0	32

Fat/Sat Fat (g)	Chol (mg)	Fibre (g)	Sugars (g)	Sodium (mg)
2/t	0	0	4	98
2/1	0	t	6	31
0/0	0	0	na	8
1/t	na	0	18	0
0/0	0	0	40	15
0/0	0	0	40	15
0/0	0	0	106	39
0/0	0	0	49	45
0/0	0	0	32	26

Beverages (cont.)	Serving	Calories	Prot (g)	Carb (g)
Lemon-lime soda, w/o caffeine	1 can or bottle (12 fl. oz.)	147	0	38
Lemon-lime soda, w/ caffeine	1 can or bottle (12 fl. oz.)	147	0	38
Orange soda	1 can or bottle (12 fl. oz.)	179	0	46
Dr Pepper-type, w/ caffeine	1 can or bottle (12 fl. oz.)	151	0	38
Root beer	1 can or bottle (12 fl. oz.)	152	0	39

Fat/Sat Fat (g)	Chol (mg)	Fibre (g)	Sugars (g)	Sodium (mg)
0/0	0	0	38	40
0/0	0	0	38	40
0/0	0	0	na	45
t/t	0	0	na	37
0/0	0	0	na	48

LOW-RESPONSE COST, LOW-YIELD FOODS: BREAD PRODUCTS, SAVOURY BISCUITS, AND MUFFINS

Food	Serving	Calories	Prot (g)	Carb (g)
Bread Products				
Bread, white	1 slice	67	2	13
French baguette	1 slice	77	3	16
French rolls	1 roll	105	3	19
Hamburger buns	1 serving	117	3.5	22
Hot dog roll	1 roll	123	4	22
Rolls (includes brown-and-serve)	1 roll (1 oz.)	84	2	14
Taco shells, corn, fried	1 medium (13 cm/5" dia)	98	1.5	13
Tortillas, ready-to-bake or -fry, white flour	1 tortilla (18–20 cm/ 7–8" dia.)	150	4	25.5
Tortillas, ready-to-bake or -fry, white flour	1 tortilla (25 cm/ 10" dia.)	228	6	39
Savoury Biscuits				
Butter-type	1 serving	79	1	10
Matzo, plain	1 matzo	111	3	23

Fat/Sat Fat (g)	Chol (mg)	Fibre (g)	Sugars (g)	Sodium (mg)
1/0	0	0	t	7
1/0	0	t	t	192
2/t	0	1	na	231
2/t	na	1	5	256
2/t	0	1	na	241
2/t	0	1	na	146
5/1	na	2	na	77
3/1	0	1.5	na	220
5/1	0	2	na	335
4/1	0	t	1	124
t/t	0	1	na	1

Bread Products (cont.)	Serving	Calories	Prot (g)	Carb (g)
Muffins				
Blueberry, American-style, commercially prepared	1 large	385	8	67
Blueberry, American-style, commercially prepared	1 medium	313	6	54
Blueberry, American-style, commercially prepared	1 small	183	4	32
Blueberry, American-style, commercially prepared	1 mini	47	1	8
Blueberry, American-style, prepared from recipe, made w/ semi-skimmed milk	1 muffin	162	4	23
Plain, American-style, prepared from recipe, made w/ semi-skimmed milk	1 muffin	169	4	24
Muffin, plain	1 muffin	134	4	26
Muffin, plain	1 muffin	133	4	26
Scone	1 scone (2 oz.)	175	3.5	25.8

Fat/Sat Fat (g)	Chol (mg)	Fibre (g)	Sugars (g)	Sodium (mg)
9/2	42	4	na	621
7/1.5	34	3	na	505
4/1	20	2	na	295
1/t	5	t	na	76
6/1	21	na	na	251
7/1	22	1.5	na	266
1/t	0	1.5	na	264
1/t	0	1.5	na	262
7/1.8	3	0.9	2.9	403

LOW-RESPONSE COST, LOW-YIELD FOODS: CAKES AND PIES

Food	Serving	Calories	Prot (g)	Carb (g)
Cakes				
Angel food cake, commercially prepared	1 piece (1/12 of 12 oz. cake)	72	2	16
Chocolate cake, commercially prepared	1 piece (1/8 of 18 oz. cake)	235	3	35
Chocolate snack cake, crème filling	1 serving	368	3	45
Fairy cakes, chocolate, w/ frosting, low-fat	1 cake	131	2	29
Fruitcake, commercially prepared	1 piece	139	1	26
Gingerbread cake, prepared from recipe	1 piece	263	3	36
Pineapple upside-down cake, prepared from recipe	1 piece (1/8 of 8" square)	367	4	58
Pound cake, commercially prepared, butter	1 piece (1/12 of 12 oz. cake)	109	1.5	14

Fat/Sat Fat (g)	Chol (mg)	Fibre (g)	Sugars (g)	Sodium (mg)
t/t	0	t	na	210
10.5/3	27	2	na	214
19/11	14	2	32	241
1.5/t	0	2	na	178
4/t	2	2	na	116
12/3	24	na	na	242
14/3	25	1	na	367
5.5/3	62	t	na	111

Cakes & Pies (cont.)	Serving	Calories	Prot (g)	Carb (g)
Pound cake, commercially prepared, other than all butter, unenriched	1 piece (1/12 of 12 oz. cake)	109	1.5	15
Shortcake, biscuit-type, prepared from recipe	2 oz.	196	3.5	27.5
Sponge cake, commercially prepared	1 piece (1/12 of 16 oz. cake)	110	2	23
Sponge cake, prepared from recipe	1 piece (1/12 of 16 oz. cake)	187	5	36

Pies

	Serving	Calories	Prot (g)	Carb (g)
Apple, frozen, ready-to-bake	1 serving	292	3	41
Apple, commercially prepared	1 piece (1/8 of 23 cm/ 9" dia)	296	2	42.5
Apple, commercially prepared	1 piece (1/6 of 20 cm/ 8" dia)	277	2	40
Apple, prepared from recipe	1 piece (1/8 of 23 cm/ 9" dia)	411	4	57.5

Fat/Sat Fat (g)	Chol (mg)	Fibre (g)	Sugars (g)	Sodium (mg)
5/1	16	t	na	112
8/2	2	na	na	287
1/t	39	t	na	93
3/1	107	na	na	144

Fat/Sat Fat (g)	Chol (mg)	Fibre (g)	Sugars (g)	Sodium (mg)
13/6	9	1	26	361
14/5	0	2	na	333
13/4	0	2	na	311
19/5	0	na	na	327

Cakes & Pies (cont.)	Serving	Calories	Prot (g)	Carb (g)
Blueberry, commercially prepared	1 piece (⅙ of 20 cm/ 8" dia)	271	2	41
Blueberry, prepared from recipe	1 piece (⅛ of 23 cm/ 9" dia)	360	4	49
Cherry, commercially prepared	1 piece (⅛ of 23 cm/ 9" dia)	325	2.5	50
Cherry, commercially prepared	1 piece (⅙ of 20 cm/ 8" dia)	304	2	46.5
Cherry, prepared from recipe	1 piece (⅛ of 23 cm/ 9" dia)	486	5	69
Egg custard, commercially prepared	1 piece (⅙ of 8" dia)	221	6	22
Lemon meringue, commercially prepared	1 piece (⅙ of 20 cm/ 8" dia)	303	2	53
Lemon meringue, prepared from recipe	1 piece (⅛ of 23 cm/ 9" dia)	362	5	50
Mincemeat, prepared from recipe	1 piece (⅛ of 23 cm/ 9" dia)	477	4	79

Fat/Sat Fat (g)	Chol (mg)	Fibre (g)	Sugars (g)	Sodium (mg)
12/2	0	1	na	380
17/4	0	na	na	272
14/3	0	1	na	308
13/3	0	1	na	288
22/5	0	na	na	344
12/2	35	2	na	252
10/2	51	1	na	165
16/4	67	na	na	307
18/4	0	4	na	419

Cakes & Pies (cont.)	Serving	Calories	Prot (g)	Carb (g)
Pecan, commercially prepared	1 piece (⅙ of 20 cm/ 8" dia)	452	4.5	65
Pecan, prepared from recipe	1 piece (⅛ of 23 cm/ 9" dia)	503	6	64
Pumpkin, prepared from recipe	1 piece (⅛ of 23 cm/ 9" dia)	316	7	41

Fat/Sat Fat (g)	Chol (mg)	Fibre (g)	Sugars (g)	Sodium (mg)
21/4	36	4	na	479
27/5	106	na	na	320
14/5	65	na	na	349

LOW-RESPONSE COST, LOW-YIELD FOODS: CEREALS AND CEREAL BARS

Food	Serving	Calories	Prot (g)	Carb (g)
Cereals—Cold				
Apple cinnamon	¾ cup	118	2	25
Apple-flavoured cereal	I cup	117	1	27
Chocolate-flavoured crisp cereal	¾ cup	118	1	27
Chocolate-flavoured puff cereal	I cup	117	1	26
Cookie crisp-type cereal	I cup	117	1	26
Corn-based puff cereal	I cup	118	1	28
Frosted flakes	¾ cup	114	1	28
Frosted rice crisp cereal	¾ cup	114	1	27
Frosted wheat flake cereal	¾ cup	112	1.5	27
Fruit-flavoured cereal	I cup	118	1	26
Graham cracker cereal	¾ cup	112	1.5	25

Fat/Sat Fat (g)	Chol (mg)	Fibre (g)	Sugars (g)	Sodium (mg)
1.5/t	0	1	13	120
1/t	0	1	15	143
1/t	0	1	14	190
1/t	0	1	14	171
1/t	0	t	13	178
t/t	0	t	14	120
t/t	0	1	12	148
t/t	0	t	12	218
t/t	0	1	12	204
1/t	0	1	14	141
1/t	0	1	10.5	269

Cereals (cont.)	Serving	Calories	Prot (g)	Carb (g)
Honey nut-flavoured cereal	1 cup	214	4	46
Honey-roasted oat cereal	¾ cup	118	2	24.5
Oatmeal crisp w/ almonds cereal	1 cup	218	5.5	42
Oatmeal crisp w/ apples cereal	1 cup	207	5	45
Puffed rice, pre-sweetened	¾ cup	108	1	24
Waffle crisp cereal	1 cup	129	2	24
Cereal Bars				
Cereal bar, fruit	1 bar (1 oz.)	103	1	20
Cereal bar, mixed berry	1 bar (1 oz.)	104	1	20
Cereal bar, hard, almond	1 bar	119	2	15
Cereal bar, hard, chocolate chip	1 bar	105	2	17
Cereal bar, hard, peanut	1 bar (1 oz.)	136	3	18
Cereal bar, hard, plain	1 bar (1 oz.)	132	3	18

Fat/Sat Fat (g)	Chol (mg)	Fibre (g)	Sugars (g)	Sodium (mg)
3/t	0	3	na	249
2/t	0	1.5	6	193
5/1	0	4	15	237
2/t	0	4	19	253
1/0	0	0	12	158
3/t	0	t	9.5	130
2/t	0	1	na	83
2/t	0	t	9	83
6/3	0	1	na	61
4/3	0	1	na	83
6/1	0	1	na	79
5.5/1	0	1.5	na	82

Cereals (cont.)	Serving	Calories	Prot (g)	Carb (g)
Cereal bar, soft, chocolate chip w/ milk chocolate coating	1 bar (1.25 oz.)	163	2	22
Cereal bar, soft, chocolate chip w/ milk chocolate coating	1 bar (1 oz.)	130	2	18
Cereal bar, soft, chocolate chip, uncoated	1 bar (1.5 oz.)	181	3	30
Cereal bar, soft, chocolate chip, uncoated	1 bar (1 oz.)	118	2	19
Cereal bar, soft, nut and raisin, uncoated	1 bar (1 oz.)	127	2	18
Cereal bar, soft, plain, uncoated	1 bar (1 oz.)	124	2	19
Cereal bar, soft, raisin, uncoated	1 bar (1.5 oz.)	193	3	28.5
Cereal bar, soft, raisin, uncoated	1 bar (1 oz.)	125	2	18.5
Chocolate chip crisped rice bar	1 bar (1 oz.)	113	1	20

Fat/Sat Fat (g)	Chol (mg)	Fibre (g)	Sugars (g)	Sodium (mg)
9/5	2	1	na	70
7/4	1	1	na	56
7/4	0	2	na	117
5/3	0	1	na	76
6/3	0	2	na	71
5/2	0	1	na	78
8/4	0	2	na	121
5/3	0	1	na	79
4/1	0	1	na	78

LOW-RESPONSE COST, LOW-YIELD FOODS: CHEESES

Food	Serving	Calories	Prot (g)	Carb (g)
Cheeses—Full Fat				
Cheese, blue	1 oz.	100	6	1
Brie	1 oz.	95	6	t
Camembert	1 oz.	85	6	t
Caraway	1 oz.	107	7	1
Cheddar	1 oz.	114	7	t
Cream cheese	1 tbsp	51	1	0
Cottage, large or small curd, full fat	½ cup, small curd, not packed	116	14	3
Cottage, full fat w/ fruit	½ cup, not packed	140	11	15
Edam	1 oz.	101	7	t
Feta	1 oz.	75	4	1
Fontina	1 oz.	110	7	t
Goat, hard type	1 oz.	128	9	1
Goat, semi-soft type	1 oz.	103	6	1
Goat, soft type	1 oz.	76	5	t

Fat/Sat Fat (g)	Chol (mg)	Fibre (g)	Sugars (g)	Sodium (mg)
8/5	21	0	na	395
8/5	28	0	na	178
7/4	20	0	na	239
8/5	26	0	na	196
9/6	30	0	na	176
5/3	16	0	0	43
5/3	17	0	na	456
4/2	12	0	na	458
8/5	25	0	na	274
6/4	25	0	na	316
9/5	33	0	na	227
10/7	30	0	na	98
8/6	22	0	na	146
6/4	13	0	na	104

Cheeses (cont.)	Serving	Calories	Prot (g)	Carb (g)
Gouda	1 oz.	101	7	1
Gruyère	1 oz.	117	8.5	t
Monterey Jack	1 oz.	106	7	t
Mozzarella, whole milk	1 oz.	80	5.5	1
Neufchatel	1 oz.	74	3	1
Parmesan, grated	2 tbsp	46	4	t
Parmesan, hard	1 oz.	111	10	1
Port de Salut	1 oz.	100	7	t
Ricotta, whole milk	½ cup	214	14	4
Roquefort	1 oz.	105	6	t

Fat/Sat Fat (g)	Chol (mg)	Fibre (g)	Sugars (g)	Sodium (mg)
8/5	32	0	na	232
9/5	31	0	na	95
8.5/5	25	0	na	152
6/4	22	0	na	106
7/4	22	0	na	113
3/2	8	0	na	186
7/5	19	0	na	454
8/5	35	0	na	151
16/10	63	0	na	103
9/5	26	0	na	513

LOW-RESPONSE COST, LOW-YIELD FOODS: COOKIES AND BISCUITS

Food	Serving	Calories	Prot (g)	Carb (g)
Cookies and biscuits				
Apricot-filled biscuits	1 serving	100	1	16
Bourbons	1 biscuit	67	1	10
Butter biscuits, commercially prepared, unenriched	1 biscuit	23	t	3
Brownies, prepared from recipe	1 brownie (5 cm/2" square)	112	1	12
Brownies, commercially prepared	1 package, twin wrapped	247	3	39
Brownies, commercially prepared	1 brownie, large (7 cm/ 2¾" square x 2 cm/⅞")	227	3	36
Chocolate chip cookie, prepared from recipe, made w/ margarine	1 cookie, medium (6 cm/2¼" dia)	78	1	9
Chocolate chip cookie, prepared from recipe, made w/ margarine	1 bar (5 cm/2" square)	156	2	19

Fat/Sat Fat (g)	Chol (mg)	Fibre (g)	Sugars (g)	Sodium (mg)
3/1	7	t	8	80
3/1.5	7	0.2	5	20
1/.5	6	0	na	18
7/2	18	na	na	82
10/3	10	1	na	190
9/2	10	1	na	175
5/1	5	t	na	58
9/3	10	1	na	116

Cookies (cont.)	Serving	Calories	Prot (g)	Carb (g)
Chocolate chip cookie, prepared from recipe, made w/ butter	I cookie, medium (6 cm/2¼" dia)	78	I	9
Chocolate chip cookie, commercially prepared, soft type	I cookie	69	I	9
Chocolate wafers	I wafer	26	t	4
Coconut macaroons, prepared from recipe	I biscuit, medium (5 cm/2" dia)	97	I	17
Custard creams	I biscuit	58	0.7	8.7
Fig bars	I bar	56	I	II
Fortune cookie	I cookie	30	t	7
Fudge, cake-type	I piece	73	I	16
Ginger biscuits	I biscuit	29	t	5
Ginger biscuits	I large (9–10 cm/ 3½"–4" dia)	133	2	25
Hob Nobs	I biscuit	68	I	9
Jammie Dodger	I biscuit	88	I	15
Oatmeal biscuits	I serving	111	2	17

Fat/Sat Fat (g)	Chol (mg)	Fibre (g)	Sugars (g)	Sodium (mg)
5/2	11	na	na	55
4/1	0	t	na	49
1/t	0	t	na	35
3/3	0	t	na	59
2.5/1.3	6	0.2	4	17
1/t	0	1	na	56
t/t	0	t	4	22
1/t	0	1	na	40
1/t	0	t	na	46
3/1	0	1	na	209
3/1.3	3	0.5	3.6	76
3.5/1.4	5	0.3	6	46
4/1	4	1	9	114

Cookies (cont.)	Serving	Calories	Prot (g)	Carb (g)
Oatmeal biscuits, prepared from recipe, w/o raisins	1 biscuit (7 cm/2⅝" dia)	67	1	10
Oatmeal biscuits, prepared from recipe, w/ raisins	1 biscuit (7 cm/2⅝" dia)	65	1	10
Oatmeal biscuits, commercially prepared, soft-type	1 biscuit	61	1	10
Oatmeal biscuits, commercially prepared, regular	1 biscuit, large	81	1	12
Oatmeal biscuits, commercially prepared, regular	1 biscuit, big (9–10 cm/ 3½"–4" dia)	113	2	17
Oatmeal raisin biscuit	1 serving	107	1	17
Raisin biscuits, soft-type	1 biscuit	60	1	10
Rich Tea	1 biscuit	43	0.7	7.5
Shortbread biscuit, commercially prepared, plain	1 biscuit (4 cm/1⅝" square)	40	t	5
Strawberry-filled biscuit	1 serving	100	1	16

Fat/Sat Fat (g)	Chol (mg)	Fibre (g)	Sugars (g)	Sodium (mg)
3/1	5	na	na	90
2/t	5	na	na	81
2/1	1	t	na	52
3/1	0	1	na	69
5/1	0	1	na	96
4/1	3	1	9	98
2/1	0	t	na	51
1.3/0.6	3	0.2	2	41
2/t	2	t	na	36
3/1	7	t	8	84

Cookies (cont.)	Serving	Calories	Prot (g)	Carb (g)
Sugar wafer w/ crème filling	1 wafer, small (60 x 19 x 6 mm/ 2½ x ¾ x ¼")	18	t	2
Sugar wafer w/ crème filling	1 wafer, large (90 x 25 x 13 mm/ 3½ x 1 x ½")	46	t	6
Vanilla wafer	1 wafer	28	t	4

Fat/Sat Fat (g)	Chol (mg)	Fibre (g)	Sugars (g)	Sodium (mg)
1/t	0	0	na	5
2/t	0	t	na	13
1/t	0	t	na	18

LOW-RESPONSE COST, LOW-YIELD FOODS: DINNERS, CANNED AND FROZEN

Food	Serving	Calories	Prot (g)	Carb (g)
Dinners Canned				
Beef ravioli in tomato and meat sauce	1 serving	229	8	37
Beef ravioli in tomato and meat sauce, mini ravioli	1 serving	239	9	41
Beef stew	1 serving	218	11	16
Chow mein, no noodles or rice	2 cups	160	16	12
Macaroni w/ beef in tomato sauce	1 serving	184	8	31
Macaroni and cheese	1 serving	199	7.5	29
Spaghetti and meatballs in tomato sauce	1 serving	250	9	34

Fat/Sat Fat (g)	Chol (mg)	Fibre (g)	Sugars (g)	Sodium (mg)
5/2	15	4	5	1174
5/2	18	3	5	1197
12/5	37	3.5	2	947
7/3	40	6	4	2380
3/1	17	3	5	799
6/3	8	3	2	1058
9/4	22	2	7	941

LOW-RESPONSE COST, LOW-YIELD FOODS: DOUGHNUTS AND PASTRIES

Food	Serving	Calories	Prot (g)	Carb (g)
Doughnuts				
Plain, sugared or glazed	1 doughnut, medium (8 cm/3" dia)	192	2	23
Plain, chocolate-coated or frosted	1 doughnut, large (9 cm/3½ " dia)	270	3	27
Plain, chocolate-coated or frosted	1 doughnut, medium (8 cm/3" dia)	204	2	21
Plain, chocolate-coated or frosted	1 doughnut (5 cm/2" dia)	133	1	13
Plain, unsugared, old fashioned	1 doughnut stick	219	3	26
Plain, unsugared, old fashioned	1 doughnut, large (10 cm/4" dia)	299	3.5	35
Plain, unsugared, old fashioned	1 doughnut, mini (4 cm/1½" dia) or doughnut hole	59	1	7

Fat/Sat Fat (g)	Chol (mg)	Fibre (g)	Sugars (g)	Sodium (mg)
10/3	14	1	na	181
18/5	35	1	na	245
13/3	26	1	na	184
9/2	17	1	na	120
12/2	19	1	na	284
16/2.5	26	1	na	388
3/t	5	t	na	76

Doughnuts (cont.)	Serving	Calories	Prot (g)	Carb (g)
Plain, unsugared, old fashioned	1 doughnut, medium (8 cm/3¼" dia)	198	2	23
Plain, unsugared, old fashioned	1 doughnut, long type (twist) (11 cm/4½" long)	219	3	26
Chocolate, sugared or glazed	1 doughnut, medium (8 cm/3" dia)	175	2	24
Chocolate, sugared or glazed	1 doughnut, (9 cm/3¾" dia)	250	3	34
Yeast-leavened, w/ crème filling	1 doughnut oval (9 x 6 cm/3½ x 2½")	307	5	25.5
Yeast-leavened, w/ jelly filling	1 doughnut oval (9 x 6 cm/3½ x 2½")	289	5	33
Doughnut stick, cake-type, plain	1 doughnut stick	219	3	26
Doughnut stick, yeast-leavened, glazed, enriched	1 doughnut stick	226	3.5	25

Fat/Sat Fat (g)	Chol (mg)	Fibre (g)	Sugars (g)	Sodium (mg)
11/2	17	1	na	257
12/2	19	1	na	284
8/2	24	1	na	143
12/3	34	1	na	204
21/5	20	1	na	263
16/4	22	1	na	249
12/2	19	1	na	284
13/3	3	1	na	192

Doughnuts (cont.)	Serving	Calories	Prot (g)	Carb (g)
Doughnut twist, yeast-leavened, glazed, enriched	1 doughnut twist (11 cm/ 4½" lg)	219	3	26
Doughnut hole, yeast-leavened, glazed, enriched	1 doughnut hole	52	1	6

Pastries

	Serving	Calories	Prot (g)	Carb (g)
Cream puffs, prepared from recipe	1 cream puff	335	9	30
Coffeecake, cinnamon w/ crumb topping, commercially prepared	1 piece (⅑ of 20 oz. cake)	263	4	29
Coffeecake, fruit	1 piece (⅛ cake)	156	3	26
Croissant, apple	1 croissant, medium	145	4	21
Croissant, butter	1 croissant, large	272	5.5	31
Croissant, butter	1 croissant, medium	231	5	26
Croissant, butter	1 croissant, small	171	3	19

Fat/Sat Fat (g)	Chol (mg)	Fibre (g)	Sugars (g)	Sodium (mg)
12/2	19	1	na	284
3/1	1	t	na	44
20/5	174	t	na	443
15/4	20	1	na	221
5/1	4	1	na	193
5/3	18	1	na	156
14/8	45	2	na	498
12/7	38	1.5	na	424
9/5	28	1	na	312

Doughnuts (cont.)	Serving	Calories	Prot (g)	Carb (g)
Croissant, butter	1 croissant, mini	114	2	13
Danish pastry, cheese	1 pastry	266	6	26
Danish pastry, cinnamon	1 pastry, large (18 cm/ 7" dia.)	572	10	63
Danish pastry, cinnamon	1 pastry, (11 cm/4¼" dia)	262	4.5	29
Danish pastry, cinnamon	1 pastry, small or frozen (8 cm/ 3" dia)	141	2	16
Danish pastry, fruit	1 pastry, large (18 cm/ 7" dia)	527	8	68
Danish pastry, fruit	1 pastry (11 cm/4¼" dia)	263	4	34
Danish pastry, fruit	1 pastry, small or frozen (8 cm/ 3" dia)	130	2	17
Danish pastry, nut	1 pastry (11 cm/4¼" dia)	280	5	30

Fat/Sat Fat (g)	Chol (mg)	Fibre (g)	Sugars (g)	Sodium (mg)
6/3	19	1	na	208
15.5/5	11	1	na	320
32/8	30	2	na	527
14.5/4	14	1	na	241
8/2	7	t	na	44
26/7	162	3	na	503
13/3	81	1	na	251
6/2	40	1	na	124
16/4	30	1	na	236

Doughnuts (cont.)	Serving	Calories	Prot (g)	Carb (g)
Eclairs, custard-filled w/ chocolate glaze, prepared from recipe	1 small éclair, (9 x 5 cm/ 3½ x 2")	293	7	27
Eclairs, custard-filled w/ chocolate glaze, prepared from recipe	1 medium éclair, (13 x 5 x 4 cm/ 5 x 2 x 1¾")	262	6	24

Fat/Sat Fat (g)	Chol (mg)	Fibre (g)	Sugars (g)	Sodium (mg)
18/5	142	1	na	377
16/4	127	1	na	337

LOW-RESPONSE COST, LOW-YIELD FOODS: EGGS

Food	Serving	Calories	Prot (g)	Carb (g)
Eggs				
Fried	1 large	92	6	t
Omelette	1 large	93	6	1
Scrambled	1 large	101	7	1

Fat/Sat Fat (g)	Chol (mg)	Fibre (g)	Sugars (g)	Sodium (mg)
7/2	211	0	0	162
7/2	214	0	0	165
7/2	215	0	0	171

LOW-RESPONSE COST, LOW-YIELD FOODS: FAST FOODS

Food	Serving	Calories	Prot (g)	Carb (g)
Breakfast Foods				
Cinnamon roll	1 roll	535	9	96
Croissant with egg and cheese	1 croissant	368	13	24
Croissant with egg, cheese and bacon	1 croissant	413	16	24
Croissant with egg, cheese, and ham	1 croissant	474	19	24
Danish pastry, cinnamon	1 pastry	349	5	47
Danish pastry, fruit	1 pastry	335	5	45
Egg and cheese sandwich	1 sandwich	340	16	26
Egg, scrambled	2 eggs	199	13	2
Ham, egg, and cheese sandwich	1 sandwich	347	19	31
Muffin, with butter	1 muffin	189	5	30

Fat/Sat Fat (g)	Chol (mg)	Fibre (g)	Sugars (g)	Sodium (mg)
21/7	17	na	na	770
25/14	216	na	na	551
28/15	215	na	na	889
33.5/17.5	213	na	na	1081
17/3.5	27	na	na	326
16/3	19	na	na	333
19/7	291	na	na	804
15/6	400	0	na	211
16/7	246	na	na	1005
6/2	13	na	na	386

Fast Foods (cont.)	Serving	Calories	Prot (g)	Carb (g)
Muffin with cheese and sausage	1 muffin	393	15	29
Muffin with egg, cheese and sausage	1 muffin	487	22	31
Pancakes with butter and syrup	2 cakes	520	8	91
Burgers				
Bacon cheeseburger, ⅓ lb.	1 sandwich	800	39	41
Bacon cheeseburger, ⅔ lb.	1 sandwich	1148	63	42
Cheeseburger, large double burger, w/ condiments	1 sandwich	704	38	40
Cheeseburger, large, single burger, w/ condiments	1 sandwich	563	28	38
Cheeseburger, regular, double burger, plain	1 sandwich	461	22	44
Cheeseburger, regular, double burger, w/ condiments	1 sandwich	650	30	53

Fat/Sat Fat (g)	Chol (mg)	Fibre (g)	Sugars (g)	Sodium (mg)
24/10	59	1.5	na	1036
31/12	274	na	na	1135
14/6	58	na	na	1104
55/18	120	na	na	1413
82/31	198	na	na	2042
44/18	142	na	na	1148
33/15	88	na	na	1108
22/9.5	80	na	na	891
35/13	93	na	na	921

Fast Foods (cont.)	Serving	Calories	Prot (g)	Carb (g)
Cheeseburger, regular, single burger, w/ condiments	1 sandwich	295	16	27
Cheeseburger, triple burger, plain	1 sandwich	796	56	27
Hamburger, large, double burger, w/ condiments	1 sandwich	540	34	40
Hamburger, large, single burger, w/ condiments	1 sandwich	427	23	37
Hamburger, large, triple burger, w/ condiments	1 sandwich	692	50	28.5
Hamburger, regular, double burger, plain	1 sandwich	544	30	43
Hamburger, regular, double burger, w/ condiments	1 sandwich	576	32	39
Hamburger, regular, single burger, plain	1 sandwich	275	12	30.5
Hamburger, regular, single burger, w/ condiments	1 sandwich	272	12	34

Fat/Sat Fat (g)	Chol (mg)	Fibre (g)	Sugars (g)	Sodium (mg)
14/6	37	na	na	616
51/22	161	na	na	1213
26.5/10.5	122	na	na	791
21/8	71	2	8	731
41/16	142	na	na	712
28/10	99	na	na	554
32/12	103	na	na	742
12/4	35	na	na	387
10/3.5	30	2	7	534

Fast Foods (cont.)	Serving	Calories	Prot (g)	Carb (g)
Chicken				
Chicken club sandwich	1 sandwich	470	30	47
Chicken fillet sandwich, plain	1 sandwich	515	24	39
Chicken fillet sandwich, w/ cheese	1 sandwich	632	29	41.5
Chicken pieces, breaded and fried, plain	6 pieces	319	18	15
Chicken pieces, breaded and fried, w/ barbecue sauce	6 pieces	330	17	25
Chicken pieces, breaded and fried, w/ honey	6 pieces	329	17	27
Chicken pieces, breaded and fried, w/ mustard sauce	6 pieces	322	17	21
Chicken pieces, breaded and fried, w/ sweet and sour sauce	6 pieces	346	17	29
Chicken strips	4 strips	290	29	14

Fat/Sat Fat (g)	Chol (mg)	Fibre (g)	Sugars (g)	Sodium (mg)
19/4	65	2	6	920
29/8.5	60	na	na	957
39/12	78	na	na	1238
21/5	61	0	0	513
18/5.5	61	na	na	829
18/5.5	61	na	na	537
19/6	61	na	na	790
18/5.5	61	na	na	677
13/2.5	65	1	3	730

Fast Foods (cont.)	Serving	Calories	Prot (g)	Carb (g)
Chicken wings, hot	6 pieces	443	37.5	t
Dark meat, breaded and fried	2 pieces	431	30	16
Light meat, breaded and fried	2 pieces	247	18	10
Roast chicken, Caesar-style, sandwich	1 sandwich	820	43	75

Desserts

	Serving	Calories	Prot (g)	Carb (g)
Dessert thick frost-type shakes, junior size	1 shake (6 oz.)	170	4	28
Dessert thick frost-type shakes, small size	1 shake (12 oz.)	330	8	56
Dessert thick frost-type shakes, medium size	1 shake (16 oz.)	440	11	73
Ice cream cone, chocolate, small	1 cone	240	6	37
Ice cream cone, chocolate, medium	1 cone	340	8	53
Ice cream cone, vanilla, small	1 cone	230	6	38

Fat/Sat Fat (g)	Chol (mg)	Fibre (g)	Sugars (g)	Sodium (mg)
32/8	117	t	0	114
27/7	166	na	na	755
15/4	74	na	na	487
38/9	140	5	na	2160

4/2.5	20	0	21	100
8/5	35	0	43	200
11/7	50	0	56	260
8/5	20	0	25	115
11/7	30	0	34	160
7/4.5	20	0	27	115

Fast Foods (cont.)	Serving	Calories	Prot (g)	Carb (g)
Ice cream cone, vanilla, medium	1 cone	330	8	53
Ice cream cone, vanilla, large	1 cone	410	10	65
Ice milk, vanilla, soft serve, w/ cone	1 cone	164	4	24
Malt, chocolate, small	1 malt (418 g.)	650	15	111
Malt, chocolate, medium	1 malt (567 g.)	880	19	153
Shake, chocolate, regular	1 shake (10 fl. oz.)	264	7	43
Shake, chocolate, large	1 shake (22 fl. oz.)	582	15.5	94
Shake, strawberry, regular	1 shake (10 fl. oz.)	320	10	53
Shake, strawberry, large	1 shake (22 fl. oz.)	704	21	118
Shake, vanilla, regular	1 shake (10 fl. oz.)	231	7	37
Shake, vanilla, large	1 shake (22 fl. oz.)	508	16	82
Sundae, caramel	1 sundae	304	7	49

Fat/Sat Fat (g)	Chol (mg)	Fibre (g)	Sugars (g)	Sodium (mg)
9/6	30	0	38	160
12/8	40	0	49	200
6/3.5	28	t	na	92
16/10	55	0	95	370
22/14	70	0	131	500
8/5	27	2	na	202
17/11	60	4	na	444
8/5	31	1	na	235
17/11	68	2.5	na	517
6/4	23	1	na	171
14/8.5	50	2	na	376
9/4.5	25	0	na	195

Fast Foods (cont.)	Serving	Calories	Prot (g)	Carb (g)
Sundae, hot fudge	1 sundae	284	6	48
Sundae, strawberry	1 sundae	268	6	45
Mexican Foods				
Burrito w/ beans	1 burrito	224	7	36
Burrito w/ beans and cheese	1 burrito	189	8	27
Burrito w/ beans and chilli peppers	1 burrito	206	8	29
Burrito w/ beans and meat	1 burrito	254	11	33
Burrito w/ beans, cheese, and beef	1 burrito	165	7	20
Burrito w/ beans, cheese, and chilli peppers	1 burrito	331	17	42.5
Burrito w/ beef	1 burrito	262	13	29
Burrito w/ beef and chilli peppers	1 burrito	213	11	25
Burrito w/ beef, cheese, and chilli peppers	1 burrito	316	20	32
Burrito, grilled, stuffed w/ beef	1 burrito	730	28	79

Fat/Sat Fat (g)	Chol (mg)	Fibre (g)	Sugars (g)	Sodium (mg)
9/5	21	0	na	182
8/4	21	0	na	92
7/3	2	na	na	493
6/3	14	na	na	583
7/4	16	na	na	522
9/4	24	na	na	668
7/3.5	62	na	na	495
11.5/5.5	79	na	na	1030
10/5	32	na	na	746
8/4	27	na	na	558
12/5	85	na	na	1046
33/11	55	10	7	2080

Fast Foods (cont.)	Serving	Calories	Prot (g)	Carb (g)
Burrito, grilled, stuffed w/ chicken	1 burrito	680	35	76
Burrito, grilled, stuffed w/ steak	1 burrito	680	31	76
Chilli con carne	1 cup	256	25	22
Chimichanga w/ beef	1 chimichanga	425	20	43
Chimichanga w/ beef and cheese	1 chimichanga	443	20	39
Chimichanga w/ beef and red chilli peppers	1 chimichanga	424	18	46
Chimichanga w/ beef, cheese, and red chilli peppers	1 chimichanga	364	15	38
Enchilada w/ cheese	1 enchilada	319	10	28.5
Enchilada w/ cheese and beef	1 enchilada	323	12	30
Enchilada w/ cheese, beef, and beans	1 enchilada	344	18	34
Frijoles w/ cheese	1 cup	225	11	29
Nachos w/ cheese	6–8 nachos	346	9	36

Fat/Sat Fat (g)	Chol (mg)	Fibre (g)	Sugars (g)	Sodium (mg)
26/7	70	7	6	1950
28/8	55	8	6	1940
8/3	134	na	na	1007
20/8.5	9	na	na	910
23/11	51	na	na	957
19/8	10	na	na	1169
17.5/8	50	na	na	895
19/10.5	44	na	na	784
18/9	40	na	na	1319
16/8	50	na	na	1251
8/4	37	na	na	882
19/8	18	na	na	816

Fast Foods (cont.)	Serving	Calories	Prot (g)	Carb (g)
Nachos w/ cheese and jalapeño peppers	6–8 nachos	608	17	60
Nachos w/ cheese, beans, minced beef, and peppers	6–8 nachos	569	20	56
Taco	1 taco, small	369	21	27
Taco	1 taco, large	568	32	41
Taco salad	2 cups	372	18	31
Taco salad w/ chilli con carne	2 cups	386	23	35
Tostada w/ beans and cheese	1 tostada	223	10	27
Tostada w/ beans, beef, and cheese	1 tostada	333	16	30
Tostada w/ beef, and cheese	1 tostada	315	19	23
Pizzas				
Individual, pan pizza	1 pizza	722	33	70
Regular, pepperoni	1 slice	280	13	28
Stuffed crust, pepperoni	1 slice	360	17	39

Fat/Sat Fat (g)	Chol (mg)	Fibre (g)	Sugars (g)	Sodium (mg)
34/14	84	na	na	1736
31/12	20	na	na	1800
20.5/11	56	na	na	802
32/17	87	na	na	1233
20/9	58	na	na	1016
17.5/8	7	na	na	1180
10/5	30	na	na	543
17/11	74	na	na	871
16/10	41	na	na	897
34/12	66	6	3	1760
13/6	20	2	2	790
16/7	30	3	2	1120

Fast Foods (cont.)	Serving	Calories	Prot (g)	Carb (g)
Thin crust, cheese	1 slice	400	19	41
Thin crust, pepperoni	1 slice	190	9	21

Sandwiches, other

	Serving	Calories	Prot (g)	Carb (g)
Hot dog, plain	1 sandwich	242	10	18
Hot dog w/ chilli	1 sandwich	296	14	31
Roast beef sandwich, plain	1 sandwich	346	21.5	33
Roast beef sandwich w/ Cheddar	1 sandwich	480	23	43
Roast beef sandwich, giant-size	1 sandwich (8 oz.)	480	32	41
Roast turkey sandwich w/ bacon and ranch dressing	1 sandwich	880	48	74
Ham and cheese sandwich	1 sandwich	352	21	33
Submarine sandwich w/ sliced meats	1 sandwich	456	22	51
Submarine sandwich w/ sliced meats, double meat	1 sandwich	580	31	49

Fat/Sat Fat (g)	Chol (mg)	Fibre (g)	Sugars (g)	Sodium (mg)
19/9	37	2	5	992
9/4	15	2	1	610

Fat/Sat Fat (g)	Chol (mg)	Fibre (g)	Sugars (g)	Sodium (mg)
15/5	44	na	na	670
13/5	51	na	na	480
14/4	51	na	na	792
24/8	90	2	na	1240
23/10	110	3	na	1440
44/10	155	5	na	2320
15/6	58	na	na	771
19/7	36	na	na	1651
32/11	105	4	7	2540

Fast Foods (cont.)	Serving	Calories	Prot (g)	Carb (g)
Submarine sandwich w/ meatballs, double meat	1 sandwich	780	35	61
Submarine sandwich w/ roast beef	1 sandwich	410	29	44
Submarine sandwich w/ tuna salad	1 sandwich	584	30	55
Seafood				
Battered fish	1 piece	230	11	16
Clams, breaded and fried	1 cup	601	17	52
Fish sandwich w/ tartar sauce	1 sandwich	431	17	41
Fish sandwich w/ tartar sauce and cheese	1 sandwich	523	21	48
Oysters, battered or breaded, fried	6 oysters	368	13	40
Prawns, breaded and fried	6 prawns	454	19	40
Scallops, breaded and fried	6 scallops	386	16	38

Fat/Sat Fat (g)	Chol (mg)	Fibre (g)	Sugars (g)	Sodium (mg)
41/18	85	5	10	1760
13/7	73	na	na	845
28/5	49	na	na	1293

13/4	30	0	0	700
35/9	117	na	na	1112
23/5	55	na	na	615
29/8	68	na	na	939
18/5	108	na	na	677
25/5	200	na	na	1446
19/5	108	na	na	919

Fast Foods (cont.)	Serving	Calories	Prot (g)	Carb (g)
Sides				
Chips, fried in vegetable oil	1 small serving	291	4	34
Chips, fried in vegetable oil	1 medium serving	458	6	53
Chips, fried in vegetable oil	1 large serving	578	7	67
Hash browns	½ cup	151	2	16
Mozzarella sticks	4 sticks	470	18	34
Onion rings, breaded and fried	8–9 onion rings	276	4	31
Potato, jacket, topped w/ cheese sauce	1 potato	474	15	47
Potato, jacket, topped w/ cheese sauce and bacon	1 potato	451	18	44
Potato, jacket, topped w/ cheese sauce and broccoli	1 potato	403	14	47
Potato, jacket, topped w/ cheese sauce and chilli	1 potato	482	23	56

Fat/Sat Fat (g)	Chol (mg)	Fibre (g)	Sugars (g)	Sodium (mg)
16/3	0	3	0	168
25/5	0	5	0	265
31/6.5	0	6	0	335
9/4	9	na	na	290
29/14	60	2	na	1330
15.5/7	14	na	na	430
29/11	18	na	na	382
26/10	30	na	na	972
21/8.5	20	na	na	485
22/13	32	na	na	699

Fast Foods (cont.)	Serving	Calories	Prot (g)	Carb (g)
Potato, jacket, topped w/ sour cream and chives	1 potato	393	7	50

Fat/Sat Fat (g)	Chol (mg)	Fibre (g)	Sugars (g)	Sodium (mg)
22/10	24	na	na	181

LOW-RESPONSE COST, LOW-YIELD FOODS: FATS

Fats Food	Serving	Calories	Prot (g)	Carb (g)
Fats				
Butter	1 oz.	208	0.2	0.2
Margarine, polyunsaturated	1 oz.	209	0.2	0.1
Reduced fat spread, 70% fat	1 oz.	174	0.1	0.2
Half-fat spread, 40% fat	1 oz.	102	1.4	0.5

Fat/Sat Fat (g)	Chol (mg)	Fibre (g)	Sugars (g)	Sodium (mg)
23/14.6	60	0	0.2	170
23/4.8	0.6	0	0.1	190
19.2/4.5	t	0	0.2	224
11.6/2.5	t	0	0.4	182

LOW-RESPONSE COST,
LOW-YIELD FOODS: FISH AND SHELLFISH

Food	Serving	Calories	Prot (g)	Carb (g)
Fish				
Anchovy, tinned in oil, drained	1 tin (2 oz.)	95	13	0
Catfish, breaded and fried	4 oz.	260	20.5	9
Croaker, breaded and fried	4 oz.	250	21	8.5
Fish fillet, fried, generic	1 fillet	211	13	15.5
Fish sticks, frozen, pre-heated	4 sticks	305	17.5	27
Sardine, canned in oil, drained	4 oz.	236	28	0
Shark, breaded and fried	4 oz.	258	21	7
Tuna, light, canned in oil, drained	4 oz.	225	33	0
Tuna, white, canned in oil, drained	4 oz.	211	30	0
Shellfish				
Clams, breaded and fried	4 oz.	229	16	12

Fat/Sat Fat (g)	Chol (mg)	Fibre (g)	Sugars (g)	Sodium (mg)
4/1	38	0	na	1651
15/4	92	1	na	317
14/4	95	t	na	394
11/3	31	t	na	484
14/3.5	125	0	na	652
13/2	161	0	0	573
16/4	67	0	na	138
9/2	20	0	0	401
9/2	35	0	0	449
13/3	69	na	na	413

Fish (cont.)	Serving	Calories	Prot (g)	Carb (g)
Crab cakes, fried	2 cakes	186	24	t
Oysters, breaded and fried	4 oz.	223	10	13
Prawns, breaded and fried	4 oz.	274	24	13
Scallops, breaded and fried	4 oz.	241	20	11
Squid, fried (calamari)	4 oz.	198	20	9

Fat/Sat Fat (g)	Chol (mg)	Fibre (g)	Sugars (g)	Sodium (mg)
9/2	180	0	na	396
14/4	92	na	na	473
14/2	201	t	na	390
12/3	68	na	na	520
9/2	295	0	na	347

LOW-RESPONSE COST, LOW-YIELD FOODS: FRUITS AND FRUIT DRINKS

Food	Serving	Calories	Prot (g)	Carb (g)
Fruits				
Applesauce, canned, sweetened, w/ salt	½ cup	97	t	25
Applesauce, canned, sweetened, w/o salt	½ cup	97	t	25
Apricots, canned, heavy syrup, w/o skin, solids and liquids	½ cup, whole, w/o pits	107	1	28
Apricots, canned, light syrup, w/ skin, solids and liquids	½ cup, halves	80	1	21
Blueberries, frozen, sweetened	1 cup, thawed	186	1	50
Candied fruit	100 grams	321	0	83
Cranberry sauce, canned, sweetened	½ cup	209	t	54
Fruit cocktail, canned, heavy syrup, solids and liquids	½ cup	91	t	23

Fat/Sat Fat (g)	Chol (mg)	Fibre (g)	Sugars (g)	Sodium (mg)
t/t	0	1.5	na	36
t/t	0	1.5	na	4
t/t	0	2	na	14
t/t	0	2	na	5
0/0	0	5	45	2
0/0	0	2	81	98
t/t	0	1	na	40
t/t	0	1	na	7

Fruits (cont.)	Serving	Calories	Prot (g)	Carb (g)
Fruit cocktail, canned, light syrup, solids and liquids	½ cup	69	t	18
Grapefruit sections, canned, in light syrup, solids and liquids	½ cup	76	.5	20
Peaches, canned, heavy syrup, solids and liquids	½ cup	97	1	26
Peaches, canned, light syrup, solids and liquids	½ cup, halves or slices	68	1	18
Pears, canned, heavy syrup, solids and liquids	½ cup	98	t	26
Pears, canned, light syrup, solids and liquids	½ cup, halves	72	t	19
Pineapple, canned, heavy syrup, solids and liquids	½ cup, crushed, sliced or chunks	99	t	26
Pineapple, canned, light syrup, solids and liquids	½ cup, crushed, sliced or chunks	66	t	17

Fat/Sat Fat (g)	Chol (mg)	Fibre (g)	Sugars (g)	Sodium (mg)
t/t	0	1	na	7
0/0	0	.5	19	2
t/t	0	2	na	8
t/t	0	2	na	6
t/t	0	2	na	7
t/t	0	2	na	6
t/t	0	1	na	1
t/t	0	1	na	1

Fruits (cont.)	Serving	Calories	Prot (g)	Carb (g)
Pineapple, frozen, chunks, sweetened	½ cup, chunks	104	t	27
Plums, canned, purple, light syrup, solids and liquids	½ cup, pitted	79	t	21
Prunes, canned, heavy syrup, solids and liquids	½ cup	123	1	33
Prunes, dried, stewed, w/ added sugar	½ cup, pitted	154	1	41
Rhubarb, frozen, cooked, w/ sugar	½ cup	139	t	37
Strawberries, frozen, sweetened, whole	1 cup	199	1	54

Fruit Drinks

	Serving	Calories	Prot (g)	Carb (g)
Apricot nectar, canned	1 cup (8 fl. oz.)	141	1	36
Cranberry-apple juice drink, bottled	1 cup (8 fl. oz.)	164	t	42
Cranberry-grape juice drink, bottled	1 cup (8 fl. oz.)	137	t	34
Cranberry juice cocktail, bottled	1 cup (8 fl. oz.)	144	0	36

Fat/Sat Fat (g)	Chol (mg)	Fibre (g)	Sugars (g)	Sodium (mg)
t/t	0	1	na	2
t/t	0	1	na	25
t/t	0	4	na	4
t/t	0	5	na	2
t/t	0	2	na	1
0/0	0	5	48	3

Fat/Sat Fat (g)	Chol (mg)	Fibre (g)	Sugars (g)	Sodium (mg)
t/t	0	1.5	na	8
0/0	0	t	na	5
t/t	0	t	na	7
t/t	0	t	na	5

Fruits (cont.)	Serving	Calories	Prot (g)	Carb (g)
Grape juice drink, canned	1 cup (8 fl. oz.)	125	t	32
Papaya nectar, canned	1 cup (8 fl. oz.)	143	t	36
Peach nectar, canned	1 cup (8 fl. oz.)	134	1	35
Pear nectar, canned	1 cup (8 fl. oz.)	150	t	39
Sports drink, lemon-lime flavour mix, powder	¾ scoop	58	0	15

Fat/Sat Fat (g)	Chol (mg)	Fibre (g)	Sugars (g)	Sodium (mg)
0/0	0	t	na	3
t/t	0	1.5	na	13
t/t	0	1.5	na	17
t/t	0	1.5	na	10
0/0	0	0	14	96

LOW-RESPONSE COST, LOW-YIELD FOODS: GRAINS, PASTA, AND NOODLES

Food	Serving	Calories	Prot (g)	Carb (g)
Rice				
Rice noodles, cooked	½ cup	96	1	22
White rice, short-grained, cooked	½ cup	121	2	27
White rice, long-grained, cooked	½ cup	103	2	22
White rice, long-grained, instant, cooked	½ cup	81	2	18
White rice, long-grained, parboiled, enriched, cooked	½ cup	100	2	22
Pasta and Noodles				
Fresh-refrigerated, plain	½ cup	149	6	28
Home-made, made w/o egg	½ cup	141	5	29
Macaroni, elbow	½ cup	99	3	20
Pasta, spiral	½ cup	94	3	19
Pasta, shells	½ cup	81	3	16
Spaghetti, w/ salt	½ cup	99	3	20

Fat/Sat Fat (g)	Chol (mg)	Fiber (g)	Sugars (g)	Sodium (mg)
t/t	0	1	na	17
t/t	0	na	na	0
t/t	0	t	na	1
t/t	0	.5	na	2
t/t	0	t	na	3
l/t	38	na	na	7
l/t	0	na	na	84
t/t	0	1	na	1
t/t	0	1	na	1
t/t	0	1	na	1
t/t	0	1	na	70

LOW-RESPONSE COST, LOW-YIELD FOODS: GRAVIES AND SAUCES

Food	Serving	Calories	Prot (g)	Carb (g)
Sauces				
Barbecue sauce	2 tbsp	24	1	4
Barbecue sauce, hickory smoke	2 tbsp	39	t	9
Bearnaise, dehydrated, dry	1 pkt	91	4	15
Cheese sauce, ready-to-serve	¼ cup	110	4	4
Creole sauce, ready-to-serve	¼ cup	25	1	4
Fish sauce, ready-to-serve	2 tbsp	13	2	1
Hoisin sauce, ready-to-serve	2 tbsp	70	1	14
Hollandaise, w/ butterfat, dehydrated, prepared w/ water	1 pkt	188	4	11
Jalapeño cheese sauce, ready-to-serve	¼ cup	81	2	8
Mild nacho cheese sauce, ready-to-serve	¼ cup	119	5	3

Fat/Sat Fat (g)	Chol (mg)	Fiber (g)	Sugars (g)	Sodium (mg)
1/t	0	t	na	265
t/t	0	t	7	418
2/0	0	0	na	847
8/4	18	t	t	522
1/t	0	1	3	339
0/0	0	0	na	2779
1/t	1	1	na	517
16/9	41	1	3	1232
5/2	6	0	t	571
10/4	20	.5	0	492

Gravies (cont.)	Serving	Calories	Prot (g)	Carb (g)
Nacho cheese sauce, ready-to-serve	¼ cup	128	5	4
Nacho cheese sauce, w/ jalapeño peppers, mild, ready-to-serve	¼ cup	122	1	7
Plum sauce, ready-to-serve	2 tbsp	70	t	16
Stir-fry sauce, ready-to-serve	1 tbsp	16	t	2
Sweet and sour sauce, dry	1 pkt	222	1	55
Sweet and sour glaze, ready-to-serve	2 tbsp	51	t	12
Sweet and sour sauce, ready-to-serve	2 tbsp	40	t	8
Tartar sauce	1 tbsp	74	t	2
White sauce, home-made, thin	¼ cup	66	2	5
White sauce, home-made, medium	¼ cup	92	2	6
White sauce, home-made, thick	¼ cup	116	2	7

Fat/Sat Fat (g)	Chol (mg)	Fiber (g)	Sugars (g)	Sodium (mg)
10/6	29	t	t	580
10/3	4	t	2	551
t/t	0	t	na	204
1/t	0	0	1	233
0/0	0	1	na	587
t/t	0	0	8	229
1/t	0	t	7	116
8/1	6	na	na	103
4/1	5	t	na	205
7/2	4	t	na	221
9/2	4	t	na	233

LOW-RESPONSE COST,
LOW-YIELD FOODS: ICE CREAM

Food	Serving	Calories	Prot (g)	Carb (g)
Ice Cream				
Cherry vanilla	½ cup	144	2	16
Chocolate	½ cup	175	2	16
Chocolate chip	½ cup	166	2	17
Chocolate/vanilla swirl	½ cup	161	3	17
Coffee	½ cup	149	3	14
French vanilla	½ cup	185	4	19
Fruit bar	1 bar	44	0	11
Frozen yogurt, chocolate, soft-serve	½ cup	115	3	18
Frozen yogurt, vanilla, soft-serve	½ cup	114	3	17
Fudge bar	1 bar	45	1	9
Ice cream sandwich	1 bar	159	3	21
Neopolitan	½ cup	150	3	17
Sorbet	½ cup	120	0	30
Strawberry	½ cup	127	2	18

Fat/Sat Fat (g)	Chol (mg)	Fiber (g)	Sugars (g)	Sodium (mg)
8/5	20	0	16	30
12/7	44	0	na	58
10/6	25	0	16	35
9/5	25	0	15	40
9/5	25	0	14	35
11/6	78	0	na	52
0/0	0	0	8	5
4/3	4	0	na	71
4/2	1	0	na	63
t/na	na	na	na	na
7/4	20	0	15	70
8/na	50	0	11	35
0/0	0	0	28	15
6/3	19	0	na	40

Ice Cream (cont.)	Serving	Calories	Prot (g)	Carb (g)
Vanilla	½ cup	259	4	24
Vanilla, soft-serve, ice milk	½ cup	164	4	24
Vanilla ice cream w/ dark chocolate coating	1 bar	166	2	12

Fat/Sat Fat (g)	Chol (mg)	Fiber (g)	Sugars (g)	Sodium (mg)
17/11	98	0	22	153
6/4	28	0	na	92
12/7	14	0	9	34

LOW-RESPONSE COST, LOW-YIELD FOODS: LAMB, VEAL, AND ORGAN MEATS

Food	Serving	Calories	Prot (g)	Carb (g)
Lamb				
Retail cuts, lean and fat, trimmed to 3 mm/⅛" fat, choice, cooked	4 oz.	307	29	0
Rib, lean and fat, trimmed to 3 mm/ ⅛" fat, choice, grilled	4 oz.	385	26	0
Rib, lean and fat, trimmed to 3 mm/ ⅛" fat, choice, roasted	4 oz.	386	25	0
Rib, lean and fat, trimmed to 6 mm/ ¼" fat, choice, grilled	4 oz.	409	25	0
Rib, lean and fat, trimmed to 6 mm/ ¼" fat, choice, roasted	4 oz.	407	24	0
Lamb, minced, grilled	4 oz.	321	28	0

Fat/Sat Fat (g)	Chol (mg)	Fiber (g)	Sugars (g)	Sodium (mg)
20/8	109	0	0	82
30/13	111	0	0	87
31/13	109	0	0	84
34/14	112	0	0	86
34/14	110	0	0	83
22/9	110	0	0	92

Lamb (cont.)	Serving	Calories	Prot (g)	Carb (g)
Veal				
Breast, point half, lean and fat, boneless, braised	4 oz.	281	32	0
Breast, whole, boneless, lean and fat, braised	4 oz.	301	31	0
Retail cuts, lean and fat, cooked	4 oz.	262	34	0
Organ Meats				
Brain, beef, simmered	4 oz.	181	13	0
Brain, beef, pan-fried	4 oz.	222	14	0
Brain, pork, braised	4 oz.	156	14	0
Giblets, fried	1 cup, chopped or diced	402	47	6
Sweetbread, braised	4 oz.	362	25	0
Tripe, raw	4 oz.	111	16	0
Tongue, beef, simmered	4 oz.	321	25	t
Tongue, pork, simmered	4 oz.	307	27	0

Fat/Sat Fat (g)	Chol (mg)	Fiber (g)	Sugars (g)	Sodium (mg)
16/6	129	0	0	75
19/7	128	0	0	74
13/5	129	0	0	99
14/3	2328	0	0	136
18/4	2261	0	0	179
11/2	2892	0	0	103
20/5	647	0	na	164
28/10	333	0	0	131
4/2	107	0	0	52
24/10	121	0	na	68
21/7	165	0	0	124

LOW-RESPONSE COST, LOW-YIELD FOODS: MILK, MILK PRODUCTS, CREAM, AND YOGURT

Food	Serving	Calories	Prot (g)	Carb (g)
Milk and Milk Products				
Chocolate milk	1 cup	208	8	26
Chocolate-flavoured beverage mix, prepared w/ whole milk	1 cup	226	9	31
Chocolate milk, prepared w/ whole milk and chocolate syrup	1 cup	257	9	36
Hot cocoa, home-made	1 cup	193	10	29
Malted drink mix, prepared w/ whole milk	1 cup	236	9	30
Milk, canned, condensed, sweetened	½ cup	491	12	83
Milk shake, chocolate	8 fl. oz.	270	7	48
Milk shake, vanilla	8 fl. oz.	254	9	40
Strawberry-flavoured beverage mix, prepared w/ whole milk	1 cup	234	8	33

Fat/Sat Fat (g)	Chol (mg)	Fibre (g)	Sugars (g)	Sodium (mg)
8/5	30	2	na	150
9/5.5	32	1	na	165
9/5	34	1	na	147
6/4	20	2	na	128
9/5	34	t	na	172
13/8	52	0	na	194
6/4	25	1	na	252
7/4	27	0	na	216
8/5	32	0	na	128

Milk (cont.)	Serving	Calories	Prot (g)	Carb (g)
Whole milk	1 cup	156	8	11
Cream				
Creamer, non-dairy, w/ hydrogenated vegetable oil and soy protein	1 tbsp	20	t	2
Creamer, non-dairy, w/ lauric acid oil and sodium caseinate	1 tbsp	20	t	2
Liquid, coffee or table	1 tbsp	29	t	1
Whipping, heavy	1 tbsp	52	t	t
Sour cream	1 tbsp	26	t	1
Yogurt				
Frozen yogurt, hard, low-fat, all flavours	½ cup	140	2.5	26
Frozen yogurt, chocolate, soft-serve	½ cup	115	3	18
Frozen yogurt, vanilla, soft-serve	½ cup	114	3	17
Fruit-flavoured, creamy style, low-fat (1% milkfat)	1 cup	232	9	45

Fat/Sat Fat (g)	Chol (mg)	Fibre (g)	Sugars (g)	Sodium (mg)
9/6	34	0	na	120

Fat/Sat Fat (g)	Chol (mg)	Fibre (g)	Sugars (g)	Sodium (mg)
2/t	0	0	na	12
2/1	0	0	na	12
3/2	10	0	na	6
6/3	21	0	na	6
3/2	5	0	na	6

Fat/Sat Fat (g)	Chol (mg)	Fibre (g)	Sugars (g)	Sodium (mg)
3/na	na	0	na	na
4/3	4	2	na	71
4/2.5	1	0	na	63
2/1	20	1	39	125

Milk (cont.)	Serving	Calories	Prot (g)	Carb (g)
Fruit-flavoured, low-fat (1% milkfat)	1 small container (4.4 oz.)	135	4	27
Fruit-flavoured, low-fat (1% milkfat)	1 cup	218	9	41
Fruit-flavoured, whole milk	1 cup	252	11	38
Plain, whole milk	1 cup	179	19	11
Yogurt fruit smoothies, bottled	1 bottle (10 fl. oz.)	270	8	52

Fat/Sat Fat (g)	Chol (mg)	Fibre (g)	Sugars (g)	Sodium (mg)
1/.5	11	t	24.5	56
2/1	20	.5	39.50	118
6/2	13	0	na	156
7/na	na	0	na	na
3.5/2	15	0	50	130

LOW-RESPONSE COST,
LOW-YIELD FOODS: NUTS AND SEED PRODUCTS

Food	Serving	Calories	Prot (g)	Carb (g)
Nuts and Seed Products				
Almonds, honey roasted	1 tbsp	53	2	2.5
Almonds, oil roasted, w/ salt	1 tbsp	60	2	2
Almonds, oil roasted, w/o salt	1 tbsp	60	2	2
Cashews, oil roasted, w/ salt	1 tbsp	47	1	2
Cashews, oil roasted, w/o salt	1 tbsp	47	1	2
Coconut cream, canned	½ cup	284	4	12
Coconut meat, dried, not sweetened	1 tbsp	94	1	3
Coconut meat, dried, sweetened, flaked, packaged	½ cup	175	1	18
Coconut meat, dried, sweetened, shredded	½ cup	233	1	22

Fat/Sat Fat (g)	Chol (mg)	Fibre (g)	Sugars (g)	Sodium (mg)
4/t	0	1	na	12
5/t	0	1	t	33
5/t	0	1	t	0
4/1	0	t	t	25
4/1	0	t	t	1
26/23	0	3	na	74
9/8	0	2	na	5
12/11	0	2	na	95
16.5/15	0	2	na	122

Nuts (cont.)	Serving	Calories	Prot (g)	Carb (g)
Coconut milk, canned	1 cup	445	5	6
Mixed nuts, oil roasted, w/ peanuts, w/ salt	1 tbsp	55	1	2
Mixed nuts, oil roasted, w/ peanuts, w/o salt	1 tbsp	55	1	2
Mixed nuts, oil roasted, w/o peanuts, w/ salt	1 tbsp	55	1	2
Mixed nuts, oil roasted, w/o peanuts, w/o salt	1 tbsp	55	1	2
Peanuts, oil roasted, w/ salt	1 tbsp	51	2	2
Peanuts, oil roasted, w/o salt	1 tbsp	51	2	2
Peanut butter chunk style, w/ salt	1 tbsp	94	4	3
Peanut butter smooth style, w/ salt	1 tbsp	95	4	3
Pecans, oil roasted, w/ salt	1 tbsp	49	1	1

Fat/Sat Fat (g)	Chol (mg)	Fibre (g)	Sugars (g)	Sodium (mg)
48/43	0	na	na	29
5/1	0	1	na	58
5/1	0	1	na	1
5/1	0	.5	na	63
5/1	0	.5	na	1
4/1	0	1	na	38
4/1	0	1	na	1
8/4	0	1	na	78
8/2	0	1	na	75
5/t	0	1	t	27

Nuts (cont.)	Serving	Calories	Prot (g)	Carb (g)
Pecans, oil roasted, w/o salt	1 tbsp	49	1	1
Sunflower seeds, oil roasted, w/ salt	1 tbsp	58	2	1
Sunflower seeds, oil roasted, w/o salt	1 tbsp	58	2	1
Trail mix, tropical	1 cup	570	9	92
Trail mix, regular, w/ chocolate chips, salted nuts and seeds	1 cup	707	21	66
Trail mix, regular, w/ chocolate chips, unsalted nuts and seeds	1 cup	707	21	66

Fat/Sat Fat (g)	Chol (mg)	Fibre (g)	Sugars (g)	Sodium (mg)
5/t	0	1	t	0
5/.5	0	1	na	57
5/.5	0	1	na	0
24/12	0	0	na	14
47/9	6	0	na	177
47/9	6	0	na	39

LOW-RESPONSE COST, LOW-YIELD FOODS: PANCAKES AND WAFFLES

Food	Serving	Calories	Prot (g)	Carb (g)
Pancakes				
Blueberry American-style pancakes, prepared from recipe	1 pancake (10 cm/4" dia)	84	2	11
Blueberry American-style pancakes, prepared from recipe	1 pancake (15 cm/6" dia)	171	5	22
Buttermilk American-style pancakes, prepared from recipe	1 pancake (10 cm/4" dia)	86	3	11
Buttermilk American-style pancakes, prepared from recipe	1 pancake (15 cm/6" dia)	175	5	22
Plain American-style pancakes, dry mix, prepared	1 pancake (10 cm/4" dia)	74	2	14
Plain American-style pancakes, dry mix, prepared	1 pancake (15 cm/6" dia)	149	4	28

Fat/Sat Fat (g)	Chol (mg)	Fibre (g)	Sugars (g)	Sodium (mg)
4/1	21	na	na	157
7/2	43	na	na	317
4/1	22	na	na	198
7/1	45	na	na	402
1/t	5	.5	na	239
2/t	9	1	na	484

Pancakes (cont.)	Serving	Calories	Prot (g)	Carb (g)
Plain American-style pancakes, prepared from recipe	1 pancake (10 cm/4" dia)	86	2	11
Plain American-style pancakes, prepared from recipe	1 pancake (15 cm/6" dia)	175	5	22

Waffles

	Serving	Calories	Prot (g)	Carb (g)
Frozen waffles	1 serving	197	5	30
Plain waffles	1 waffle (18 cm/7" dia)	218	6	25

Fat/Sat Fat (g)	Chol (mg)	Fibre (g)	Sugars (g)	Sodium (mg)
4/1	22	na	na	167
7/2	45	na	na	338

6/1	12	na	na	563
11/2	52	na	na	383

LOW-RESPONSE COST, LOW-YIELD FOODS: PIZZA

Food	Serving	Calories	Prot (g)	Carb (g)
Pizza*				
Cheese, whole pizza	1 pizza (30 cm/12" dia)	1122	61	164
Cheese, slice	1 slice	140	8	21
Cheese, meat, and vegetables, whole pizza	1 pizza (30 cm/12" dia)	1470	104	170
Cheese, meat, and vegetables, slice	1 slice	184	13	21
Cheese, sausage, pepperoni, and onions, frozen, whole pizza	1 package	1746	62	166
Cheese, sausage, pepperoni, and onions, frozen	1 serving	337	12	32
Crispy crust pepperoni, frozen, whole pizza	1 package	728	26	69
Crispy crust pepperoni, frozen	1 serving	364	13	35

* Includes values for whole pizzas, plus regular serving sizes.

Fat/Sat Fat (g)	Chol (mg)	Fibre (g)	Sugars (g)	Sodium (mg)
26/12	75	na	na	2681
3/1.5	9	0	na	336
43/12	164	na	na	3054
5/1.5	21	na	na	382
92/33	127	na	na	3653
18/6	25	na	na	704
39/8	23	na	na	1946
19/4	12	na	na	973

Pizza (cont.)	Serving	Calories	Prot (g)	Carb (g)
Deep-dish sausage pizza, frozen, whole pizza	1 package	1576	50	164
Deep-dish sausage pizza, frozen	1 serving	391	12	41
Pepperoni, frozen, whole pizza	1 package	1288	60	118
Pepperoni, frozen	1 serving	400	16	36
Pepperoni, whole pizza	1 pizza (30 cm/12" dia)	1446	81	159
Pepperoni, slice	1 slice	181	10	20
Sausage, green and red peppers, mushroom, frozen, whole pizza	1 package	1538	67	133
Sausage, green and red peppers, mushroom, frozen	1 serving	386	17	33
Sausage and mushroom pizza, frozen, whole pizza	1 package	1496	70	152
Sausage and mushroom pizza, frozen	1 serving	306	14	31

Fat/Sat Fat (g)	Chol (mg)	Fibre (g)	Sugars (g)	Sodium (mg)
80/23	63	na	na	3351
20/6	16	na	na	830
64/25	160	na	na	2440
21/7	34	2	na	879
56/18	113	na	na	2132
7/2	14	na	na	267
83/32	147	na	na	3050
21/8	37	na	na	765
67/25	129	na	na	3509
14/5	26	na	na	718

Pizza (cont.)	Serving	Calories	Prot (g)	Carb (g)
Sausage, mushrooms, and pepperoni, frozen, whole pizza	1 package	1736	69	160
Sausage, mushrooms, and pepperoni, frozen	1 serving	344	14	32
Sausage and pepperoni, frozen, whole pizza	1 package	1389	69	120
Sausage and pepperoni, frozen	1 serving	348	17	30

Fat/Sat Fat (g)	Chol (mg)	Fibre (g)	Sugars (g)	Sodium (mg)
91/31	117	na	na	3725
18/6	23	na	na	738
70/26	175	na	na	2828
17/7	44	na	na	708

LOW-RESPONSE COST,
LOW-YIELD FOODS: PORK PRODUCTS

Food	Serving	Calories	Prot (g)	Carb (g)
Bacon				
Bacon, back, unsmoked, grilled	1 rasher	37	5	0
Bacon, streaky, unsmoked, grilled	1 rasher	69	4	0
Pork				
Boston blade, roasted	4 oz.	305	26	0
Ham, cured, whole, roasted	4 oz.	275	24	0
Ham, burger, grilled	1 burger, cooked	205	8	1
Cutlet, cooked	4 oz.	284	32	0
Loin blade (chops), bone-in, lean and fat only, braised	4 oz.	366	25	0
Loin blade (chops), bone-in, lean and fat only, grilled	4 oz.	363	25	0
Loin blade (chops), bone-in, lean and fat only, pan-fried	4 oz.	388	24	0

Fat/Sat Fat (g)	Chol (mg)	Fibre (g)	Sugars (g)	Sodium (mg)
2/0.7	4.5	0	na	468
6/2	16	0	na	315
21/8	97	0	0	76
19/7	70	0	0	1345
19/7	43	0	0	638
17/6	96	0	0	64
29/11	96	0	0	62
28/11	97	0	0	79
31/12	96	0	0	76

Pork Products (cont.)	Serving	Calories	Prot (g)	Carb (g)
Loin blade (chops), bone-in, lean and fat only, roasted	4 oz.	366	27	0
Loin, country-style ribs, lean and fat only, braised	4 oz.	335	27	0
Loin, country-style ribs, lean and fat only, roasted	4 oz.	372	27	0
Minced, cooked	4 oz.	336	29	0
Shoulder, arm picnic, lean and fat only, braised	4 oz.	373	32	0
Shoulder, arm picnic, lean and fat only, roasted	4 oz.	359	27	0
Shoulder, blade roll, lean and fat only, roasted	4 oz.	325	20	t
Spareribs, cooked	4 oz.	448	33	0

Fat/Sat Fat (g)	Chol (mg)	Fibre (g)	Sugars (g)	Sodium (mg)
28/10	105	0	0	34
24/9	99	0	0	67
29/10	104	0	0	59
24/9	108	0	0	84
26/10	124	0	0	100
27/10	107	0	0	79
27/9	76	0	na	1103
34/12	137	0	0	105

LOW-RESPONSE COST,
LOW-YIELD FOODS: POULTRY PRODUCTS

Food	Serving	Calories	Prot (g)	Carb (g)
Poultry				
Chicken w/ skin, roasted	4 oz.	272	31	0
Chicken, dark meat, w/ skin, roasted	4 oz.	288	29	0
Chicken, dark meat, w/ skin, fried in batter	4 oz.	334	24	11
Chicken, dark meat, w/ skin, fried in flour	4 oz.	319	30	5
Chicken breast, meat and skin, fried in batter	½ breast	364	35	13
Chicken breast, meat and skin, fried in flour	½ breast	218	31	2
Chicken drumstick, meat and skin, fried in batter	1 drumstick, bone removed	193	16	6
Chicken drumstick, meat and skin, fried in flour	1 drumstick, bone removed	120	13	1

Fat/Sat Fat (g)	Chol (mg)	Fibre (g)	Sugars (g)	Sodium (mg)
14/4	100	0	0	92
18/5	104	0	0	100
21/6	100	na	na	330
19/5	103	na	na	100
18.5/5	119	t	na	385
9/2	87	t	na	74
11/3	62	t	na	194
7/2	44	0	na	44

Poultry (cont.)	Serving	Calories	Prot (g)	Carb (g)
Chicken wing, meat and skin, fried in batter	1 wing, bone removed	159	10	5
Chicken wing, meat and skin, fried in flour	1 wing, bone removed	103	8	1
Cornish game hens, meat and skin, roasted	½ bird	335	29	0
Duck, meat and skin, roasted	4 oz.	377	21	0
Goose, domesticated, meat and skin, roasted	4 oz.	342	28	0
Pâté de foie gras, (goose liver pâté), canned, smoked	1 tbsp	60	1	1
Turkey breast, meat and skin, roasted	4 oz.	141	25	0
Turkey dark meat, meat and skin, roasted	1 cup	309	38.5	0
Turkey leg, meat and skin, roasted	½ leg, bone removed	568	76	0

Fat/Sat Fat (g)	Chol (mg)	Fibre (g)	Sugars (g)	Sodium (mg)
11/3	39	t	na	157
7/2	26	0	na	25
23/6	169	0	0	83
32/11	94	0	0	66
25/8	102	0	0	78
6/2	20	0	na	91
4/1	47	0	0	445
16/5	125	0	0	106
27/8	232	0	0	210

Poultry (cont.)	Serving	Calories	Prot (g)	Carb (g)
Turkey light meat, meat and skin, roasted, chopped	1 cup	276	40	0
Turkey burger, battered, fried	1 burger	181	9	10
Turkey sticks, battered and fried	2 sticks	357	18	22
Turkey wing, meat and skin, roasted	1 wing, bone removed	426	51	0

Fat/Sat Fat (g)	Chol (mg)	Fibre (g)	Sugars (g)	Sodium (mg)
12/3	106	0	0	88
12/3	40	t	na	512
22/6	82	na	na	1073
23/6	151	0	0	113

LOW-RESPONSE COST,
LOW-YIELD FOODS: PUDDINGS

Food	Serving	Calories	Prot (g)	Carb (g)
Puddings				
Banana, dry mix, instant	1 portion makes ½ cup	92	0	23
Banana, ready-to-eat	1 can (5 oz.)	180	3	30
Chocolate, dry mix, instant	1 portion makes ½ cup	89	1	22
Chocolate, ready-to-eat	1 can (5 oz.)	189	4	32
Chocolate, ready-to-eat	1 snack size (4 oz.)	150	3	26
Lemon, dry mix, instant	1 portion makes ½ cup	95	0	24
Lemon, ready-to-eat	1 can (5 oz.)	178	t	36
Rice, dry mix	1 portion makes ½ cup	102	1	25
Rice, ready-to-eat	1 can (5 oz.)	231	3	31

Fat/Sat Fat (g)	Chol (mg)	Fibre (g)	Sugars (g)	Sodium (mg)
t/t	0	0	na	375
5/1	0	t	na	278
t/t	0	1	17	357
6/1	4	1	na	183
5/1	3	1	na	146
t/t	0	0	na	333
4/1	0	t	na	199
t/t	0	t	na	99
11/2	1	t	na	121

Puddings (cont.)	Serving	Calories	Prot (g)	Carb (g)
Tapioca, dry mix	1 portion makes ½ cup	85	t	22
Tapioca, ready-to-eat	1 can (5 oz.)	169	3	28
Tapioca, ready-to-eat	1 snack size (4 oz.)	134	2	22
Vanilla, dry mix, instant	1 portion makes ½ cup	92	0	23
Vanilla, ready-to-eat	1 snack size (4 oz.)	147	3	25

Fat/Sat Fat (g)	Chol (mg)	Fibre (g)	Sugars (g)	Sodium (mg)
t/t	0	0	15	110
5/1	1	t	25	226
4/1	1	t	20	180
t/t	0	0	19	360
4/1	8	t	na	153

LOW-RESPONSE COST, LOW-YIELD FOODS:
SLICED MEATS AND SAUSAGES

Food	Serving	Calories	Prot (g)	Carb (g)
Sliced Meats and Sausages				
Blood sausage	1 slice	94	4	0
Frankfurter, pork	1 frankfurter	204	10	t

Fat/Sat Fat (g)	Chol (mg)	Fibre (g)	Sugars (g)	Sodium (mg)
9/3	30	0	0	170
18/7	50	t	0	620

LOW-RESPONSE COST, LOW-YIELD FOODS:
SNACKS: CRISPS, PRETZELS, AND POPCORN

Food	Serving	Calories	Prot (g)	Carb (g)
Crisps				
Banana chips	1 oz.	147	1	16
Cheese puffs or twists	1 oz.	156	2	15
Cheese puffs or twists, low-fat	1 oz.	122	2	20
Corn chips, plain	¼ bag (7 oz.)	267	3	28
Cornnuts, plain	1 oz.	126	2	20
Crisps, barbecue-flavour	¼ bag (7 oz.)	243	4	26
Crisps, cheese-flavour	¼ bag (6 oz.)	211	4	25
Crisps, made from dried potatoes, plain	¼ can (7 oz.)	276	3	25
Crisps, made from dried potatoes, sour cream and onion flavour	¼ can (6.75 oz.)	271	3	25

Fat/Sat Fat (g)	Chol (mg)	Fibre (g)	Sugars (g)	Sodium (mg)
9/8	0	2	10	2
10/2	1	0	na	297
3/1	0	3	2	363
17/2	0	2	na	312
4/1	0	2	0	155
16/4	0	2	na	371
12/4	2	2	na	337
19/5	0	2	na	325
18/5	1	1	na	356

Snacks (cont.)	Serving	Calories	Prot (g)	Carb (g)
Crisps, plain, made w/ partially hydrogenated soybean oil, salted	¼ bag (8 oz.)	304	4	30
Crisps, plain, made w/ partially hydrogenated soybean oil, unsalted	¼ bag (8 oz.)	304	4	30
Crisps, plain, salted	¼ bag (8 oz.)	304	4	30
Crisps, plain, unsalted	¼ bag (8 oz.)	304	4	30
Crisps, reduced fat	¼ bag (6 oz.)	200	3	28
Crisps, sour cream and onion flavour	¼ bag (7 oz.)	263	4	25
Popcorn, caramel-coated w/ peanuts	⅔ cup	113	2	23
Popcorn, caramel-coated w/o peanuts	⅔ cup	122	1	22
Popcorn, oil-popped	2 cups	110	2	13
Potato sticks	1 oz.	147	2	15
Sesame sticks, wheat-based, salted	1 oz.	153	3	13

Fat/Sat Fat (g)	Chol (mg)	Fibre (g)	Sugars (g)	Sodium (mg)
20/3	0	3	na	337
20/3	0	3	na	5
20/6	0	3	na	337
20/6	0	3	na	5
9/2	0	3	na	209
17/4	3	3	na	309
2/t	0	1	na	84
4/1	1	1.5	na	58
6/1	0	2	na	194
10/3	0	1	0	71
10/2	0	1	0	420

Snacks (cont.)	Serving	Calories	Prot (g)	Carb (g)
Snack mix, original flavour	1 cup	260	6	37
Tortilla chips, taco flavour	¼ bag (8 oz.)	272	4	36
Pretzels				
Plain pretzel, hard, w/ salt	10 pretzels	229	5	48
Plain pretzel, hard, w/o salt	10 pretzels	229	5	48

Fat/Sat Fat (g)	Chol (mg)	Fibre (g)	Sugars (g)	Sodium (mg)
11/2	1	4	na	724
14/3	3	3	na	447

Fat/Sat Fat (g)	Chol (mg)	Fibre (g)	Sugars (g)	Sodium (mg)
2/t	0	2	na	1029
2/t	0	2	na	173

LOW-RESPONSE COST, LOW-YIELD FOODS: SOUPS

Food	Serving	Calories	Prot (g)	Carb (g)
Soups				
Bean w/ ham, chunky, ready-to-serve	1 cup (8 fl. oz.)	231	13	27
Beef w/ country vegetables, chunky, ready-to-serve	1 serving	153	12	16
Beef, chunky, ready-to-serve	1 cup (8 fl. oz.)	170	12	20
Chicken, chunky, ready-to-serve	1 cup (8 fl. oz.)	178	13	17
Cream of asparagus, canned, prepared w/ milk	1 cup (8 fl. oz.)	161	6	16
Cream of celery, canned, prepared w/ milk	1 cup (8 fl. oz.)	164	6	15
Cream of chicken, canned, prepared w/ milk	1 cup (8 fl. oz.)	191	7	15
Cream of mushroom, canned, prepared w/ milk	1 cup (8 fl. oz.)	203	6	15

Fat/Sat Fat (g)	Chol (mg)	Fibre (g)	Sugars (g)	Sodium (mg)
9/3	22	11	na	972
4/1	24	na	na	868
5/3	14	1	na	866
7/2	30	2	na	889
8/3	22	1	na	1042
10/4	32	1	na	1009
11/5	27	t	na	1047
14/5	20	.5	na	918

Soups (cont.)	Serving	Calories	Prot (g)	Carb (g)
Cream of vegetable, dehydrated, prepared w/ water	1 cup (8 fl. oz.)	107	2	12
Tomato, canned, prepared w/ milk	1 cup (8 fl. oz.)	161	6	22

Fat/Sat Fat (g)	Chol (mg)	Fibre (g)	Sugars (g)	Sodium (mg)
6/1	0	.5	na	1170
6/3	17	3	na	744

LOW-RESPONSE COST, LOW-YIELD FOODS: SUGARS, SWEETENERS, JAMS, AND SYRUPS

Food	Serving	Calories	Prot (g)	Carb (g)
Sugars				
Brown	1 tbsp unpacked	34	0	9
Icing	1 tbsp	29	0	7
White	1 lump (2 cubes)	19	0	5
White	1 packet	23	0	6
White	1 tbsp	49	0	13
Honey, Jams, Preserves, Jellies				
Honey, strained or extracted	1 tbsp	64	t	17
Jams and preserves	1 tbsp	56	t	14
Jams and preserves	1 packet	39	t	10
Jam, apricot	1 tbsp	48	t	13
Jam, apricot	1 packet	34	t	9
Jellies, all types	1 tbsp	54	t	13
Jellies, all types	1 packet	40	t	10
Orange marmalade	1 tbsp	49	t	13

Fat/Sat Fat (g)	Chol (mg)	Fibre (g)	Sugars (g)	Sodium (mg)
0/0	0	0	na	4
t/t	0	0	na	0
0/0	0	0	na	0
0/0	0	0	na	0
0/0	0	0	na	0
0/0	0	0	na	1
t/t	0	t	10	6
t/t	0	t	7	4
t/t	0	t	na	8
t/t	0	t	na	6
t/t	0	t	8	5
0/0	0	t	6	4
0/0	0	0	na	11

Sugars (cont.)	Serving	Calories	Prot (g)	Carb (g)
Orange marmalade	1 packet	34	t	9
Strawberry spread, all-fruit	1 tbsp	42	t	10
Syrups				
Blends, cane and 15% maple	1 tbsp	56	t	15
Blends, corn, refiner, and sugar	1 tbsp	64	0	17
Chocolate fudge-type syrup	2 tbsp	133	2	24
Fruit syrup	1 tbsp	53	0	14
Golden syrup	1 tbsp	45	0	12
Maple syrup	1 tbsp	52	0	13
Molasses	1 tbsp	58	0	15
Pancake, regular	1 tbsp	57	0	15
Pancake, w/ butter	1 tbsp	59	0	15
Pancake, w/ 2% maple	1 tbsp	53	0	14
Sorghum	1 tbsp	61	0	16

Fat/Sat Fat (g)	Chol (mg)	Fibre (g)	Sugars (g)	Sodium (mg)
0/0	0	0	na	8
0/0	0	na	8	4
t/t	0	0	na	21
0/0	0	0	na	14
3/1.5	1	1	16	131
0/0	0	0	na	7
0/0	0	0	12	41
t/t	0	0	13	2
0/0	0	0	11	7
0/0	0	0	na	17
t/t	1	0	na	20
t/t	0	0	na	12
0/0	0	0	na	2

LOW-RESPONSE COST, LOW-YIELD FOODS: SWEETS

Food	Serving	Calories	Prot (g)	Carb (g)
Sweets				
Almond and coco-nut bar	1 package (1.76 oz.)	235	2	29
Almond and coco-nut bar	1 bar, snack size	91	1	11
Butterscotch	3 pieces	63	0	14
Caramel bar	1 bar (1.25 oz.)	162	2	22
Caramel bar	1 bar (1.6 oz.)	208	3	29
Caramel	1 piece	39	t	8
Caramels in milk chocolate	1 package (1.91 oz.)	256	3	37
Caramels in milk chocolate	2 rolls (3 pieces per roll)	171	2	24.5
Caramels in milk chocolate	7 pieces	199	2	28.5
Carob bar	1 bar (3 oz.)	470	7	49
Chocolate-covered coconut bar	1 bar, snack size	92	1	11

Fat/Sat Fat (g)	Chol (mg)	Fibre (g)	Sugars (g)	Sodium (mg)
13/9	2	2.5	24	70
5/3	1	1	9	27
t/t	1	0	na	63
7/4	9	t	20	43
9.5/6	12	t	26	55
1/1	1	t	7	25
11/8	6	t	34.5	102
7.5/5	4	t	23	68
9/6	5	t	27	79
27/25	3	3	na	93
5/4	0	1	9	28

Sweets (cont.)	Serving	Calories	Prot (g)	Carb (g)
Chocolate-covered coconut bar	1 package (1.9 oz.)	258	2	31
Chocolate fudge, prepared from recipe	1 piece	70	t	13
Chocolate nougat bar	1 bar (0.8 oz)	96	1	18
Chocolate nougat bar	1 bar (1.813 oz.)	212	2	39
Chocolate nougat bar	1 bar, fun size	71	t	13
Chocolate wafer bar	1 bar, miniature (0.35 oz.)	52	1	6
Chocolate wafer bar	1 bar (1.5 oz.)	217	3	27
Chocolate wafer bar	1 bar (1.625 oz.)	238	3	30
Chocolate wafer bar	1 bar (2.8 oz.)	403	5	50
Chocolate wafer bar	1 bar (3.375 oz.)	496	6	62
Dark chocolate bar	1 bar (1.45 oz.)	218	2	24

Fat/Sat Fat (g)	Chol (mg)	Fibre (g)	Sugars (g)	Sodium (mg)
14/11	1	2	24	77
2/1	3	t	na	10
3/2	3	t	15	45
7/3	6	1	34	99
2/1	2	t	11	33
3/2	1	t	5	7
11/7	4	1	22	27
12/8	4	1	24	30
21/14	7	1.5	41	51
26/17	9	2	50	62
13/8	2	3	20	2

Sweets (cont.)	Serving	Calories	Prot (g)	Carb (g)
Dark chocolate bar	1 bar (2.6 oz.)	388	4	43
Dinner mints	1 piece	29	t	6
Dinner mints	5 pieces	147	1	31
Fruit chews	1 package, fun size	166	t	35
Fruit chews	1 package (2.07 oz.)	234	t	50
Fruit chews	1 serving	158	t	34
Gumdrops	10 gumdrops	139	0	36
Gumdrops	1 cup of gumdrops	703	0	180
Jelly beans	10 small	40	0	10
Jelly beans	10 large (1 oz.)	103	0	26
Marshmallows, miniature	10 pieces	22	t	6
Marshmallows, miniature	1 cup	159	1	41
Marshmallows, regular	1 piece	23	t	6

Fat/Sat Fat (g)	Chol (mg)	Fibre (g)	Sugars (g)	Sodium (mg)
24/14	4	5	35	4
1/1	0	t	na	1
6/3	0	1	na	5
3/t	0	0	28	24
5/1	0	0	39	33
3/t	0	0	27	22
0/0	0	0	na	16
0/0	0	0	na	80
t/t	0	0	na	3
t/t	0	0	na	7
t/t	0	0	4	3
t/t	0	0	28	24
t/t	0	0	4	3

Sweets (cont.)	Serving	Calories	Prot (g)	Carb (g)
Milk chocolate-coated peanuts	10 pieces	208	5	20
Milk chocolate-coated peanuts	1 cup	773	20	74
Milk chocolate-coated raisins	10 pieces	39	t	7
Milk chocolate-coated raisins	1 cup	702	7	123
Milk chocolate bar, miniature	1 bar	36	t	4
Milk chocolate bar	1 bar (1.55 oz.)	226	3	26
Milk chocolate bar w/ almonds	1 bar (1.45 oz.)	216	4	22
Milk chocolate bar w/ almonds	1 bar (1.55 oz.)	231	4	23
Milk chocolate bar w/ rice cereal	1 bar, miniature	50	1	6
Milk chocolate bar w/ rice cereal	1 bar (1.4 oz.)	198	2.5	25
Milk chocolate bar w/ rice cereal	1 bar (1.45 oz.)	223	3	28.5
Milk chocolate bar w/ rice cereal	1 bar (1.55 oz.)	218	3	28

Fat/Sat Fat (g)	Chol (mg)	Fibre (g)	Sugars (g)	Sodium (mg)
13/6	4	2	na	16
50/22	13	7	na	61
1.5/t	0	t	6	4
27/16	5	8	112	65
2/1	2	t	na	6
14/8	10	1.5	na	36
14/7	8	2.5	18	30
15/7	8	3	19	33
3/1.5	2	t	5.5	15
11/6	8	1	22	58
12/7	9	1	25	65
12/7	8	1	24	64

Sweets (cont.)	Serving	Calories	Prot (g)	Carb (g)
Milk chocolate bar w/ rice cereal	1 bar (1.65 oz.)	233	3	30
Peanut bar	1 bar (1.4 oz.)	209	6	19
Peanut bar	1 bar (1.6 oz.)	235	7	21
Peanut chocolate sweets	1 cup	877	16	103
Peanut chocolate sweets	1 package (1.67 oz.)	243	4	28
Peanut chocolate sweets	1 package (1.74 oz.)	253	5	30
Plain chocolate sweets	1 cup	1023	9	148
Plain chocolate sweets	1 box (1.48 oz.)	207	2	30
Plain chocolate sweets	1 package (1.69 oz.)	236	2	34
Peppermints	3 pieces	59	0	15
Semi-sweet chocolate	1 cup chips (6 oz. pkg)	805	7	106
Semi-sweet chocolate	1 cup of mini chips	829	7	109

Fat/Sat Fat (g)	Chol (mg)	Fibre (g)	Sugars (g)	Sodium (mg)
12/7	9	1.5	26	68
13/2	0	2	17	62
15/2	0	3	19	70
45/18	15	6	86	82
12/5	4	2	24	23
13/5	4	2	25	24
44/27	29	5	132	127
9/4.5	6	1	27	26
10/6	7	1	30.5	29
t/t	na	na	9	6
50/30	0	10	95.5	18
52/31	0	10	98	19

Sweets (cont.)	Serving	Calories	Prot (g)	Carb (g)
Semi-sweet chocolate	1 oz. or 60 pieces	136	1	18
Toffee bar	1 bar (1.4 oz.)	209	1	24
Sugar-coated almonds	6 pieces	96	2	15
Sweet chocolate bar	1 bar (1.45 oz.)	207	2	24

Fat/Sat Fat (g)	Chol (mg)	Fibre (g)	Sugars (g)	Sodium (mg)
8.5/5	0	2	16	3
12.5/7	21	t	23	124
4/t	0	1	na	4
14/8	0	2	na	7

LOW-RESPONSE COST, LOW-YIELD FOODS: VEGETABLES AND VEGETABLE PRODUCTS

Food	Serving	Calories	Prot (g)	Carb (g)
Vegetables				
Beans, baked, canned, w/ frankfurters	½ cup	184	9	20
Beans, baked, canned, w/ pork	½ cup	134	7	25
Beans, baked, canned, w/ pork and tomato sauce	½ cup	124	7	25
Beans, baked, canned, plain or vegetarian	½ cup	118	6	26
Broccoli in cheese-flavoured sauce, frozen	1 cup	113	4	15
Onion rings, breaded, par-fried, frozen, prepared, heated in oven	1 cup	195	3	18
Potatoes, au gratin, home-prepared from recipe using butter	1 cup	323	12	28

Fat/Sat Fat (g)	Chol (mg)	Fibre (g)	Sugars (g)	Sodium (mg)
9/3	8	9	na	557
2/1	9	7	na	524
1/t	9	6	na	557
t/t	0	6	na	504
4/1	na	0	na	806
13/4	0	1	na	180
19/12	56	4	na	1061

Vegetables (cont.)	Serving	Calories	Prot (g)	Carb (g)
Potatoes, au gratin, home-prepared from recipe using margarine	1 cup	323	12	28
Potatoes, au gratin, dry mix, prepared w/ water, whole milk and butter	0.17 package (5.5 oz.)	130	3	18
Potatoes, chipped, frozen, home-prepared, heated in oven, w/ salt	20 chips	200	3	31
Potatoes, chipped, frozen, home-prepared, heated in oven, w/o salt	15 chips	150	2	23
Potatoes, chipped, frozen, home-prepared, heated in oven, w/ salt	15 chips	150	2	23
Potatoes, chipped, frozen, home-prepared, heated in oven, w/ salt	20 chips	200	4	32
Potatoes, hash browns, frozen, plain, prepared	1 hash brown, oval (8 x 4 x 1 cm/3 x 1½ x ½")	63	1	8

Fat/Sat Fat (g)	Chol (mg)	Fibre (g)	Sugars (g)	Sodium (mg)
18/8	37	4	na	1061
6/4	21	1	na	612
8/1	0	3	na	266
6/1	0	2	na	23
6/1	0	2	na	200
8/2	0	4	na	266
3/1	0	1	na	10

Vegetables (cont.)	Serving	Calories	Prot (g)	Carb (g)
Potatoes, hash browns, home-prepared	1 cup	326	4	33
Potatoes, mashed, dehydrated, prepared from flakes w/o milk, whole milk and butter added	½ cup	119	2	16
Potatoes, mashed, dehydrated, prepared from granules w/ milk, water and margarine added	½ cup	83	2	14
Potatoes, mashed, dehydrated, prepared from granules w/o milk, whole milk and butter added	½ cup	113	2	15
Potatoes, mashed, home-prepared, whole milk added	½ cup	81	2	18
Potatoes, mashed, home-prepared, whole milk and butter added	½ cup	111	2	18

Fat/Sat Fat (g)	Chol (mg)	Fibre (g)	Sugars (g)	Sodium (mg)
22/8	0	3	na	37
6/4	15	2	na	349
2/1	2	2	na	246
5/3	15	2	na	270
1/t	2	2	na	318
4/3	13	2	na	310

Vegetables (cont.)	Serving	Calories	Prot (g)	Carb (g)
Potatoes, mashed, home-prepared, whole milk and margarine added	½ cup	111	2	18
Potato puffs, frozen, prepared	1 cup	284	4	39
Potato salad, home-prepared	1 cup	357	7	28
Potatoes, scalloped, home-prepared w/ butter	½ cup	105	4	13
Potatoes, scalloped, home-prepared w/ margarine	½ cup	105	4	13
Potatoes, scalloped, dry mix, prepared w/ water, whole milk and butter	0.17 package (5.5 oz.)	130	3	18
Potato wedges, frozen	½ cup	123	3	26
Spinach, creamed, frozen	1 serving	169	3	9
Spinach soufflé, home-prepared	1 cup	219	11	3

Fat/Sat Fat (g)	Chol (mg)	Fibre (g)	Sugars (g)	Sodium (mg)
4/1	2	2	na	310
14/7	0	4	na	955
20/4	170	3	na	1322
5/3	15	2	na	410
5/2	7	2	na	410
6/4	15	2	na	476
2/t	0	2	na	49
13/4	16	2	na	335
18/7	184	0	na	763

Vegetables (cont.)	Serving	Calories	Prot (g)	Carb (g)
Sweet potato, candied, home-prepared	1 potato (6 x 5 cm/ 2½ x 2" dia.)	144	1	29
Tomatoes, sun-dried, packed in oil, drained	1 cup	234	6	26

Fat/Sat Fat (g)	Chol (mg)	Fibre (g)	Sugars (g)	Sodium (mg)
3/1	8	3	na	74
15/2	0	6	na	293

METRIC CONVERSION CHARTS

WEIGHT
Multiply ounces by 28.35 to get grams or use the following approximations for grams:

Cups and Spoons	Ounces	Metric Equivalents
1 tbsp.	3 tsp.	
2 tbsp.	1 oz.	25 g
4 tbsp. = ¼ cup	2 oz.	55 g
6 tbsp.	3 oz.	85 g
8 tbsp. = ½ cup	4 oz.	115 g
	5 oz.	140 g
¾ cup	6 oz.	170 g
	7 oz.	200 g
1 cup = ½ lb	8 oz.	225 g
	9 oz.	255 g
	10 oz.	280 g
1½ cups	12 oz.	340 g
2 cups = 1 lb	16 oz.	450 g

VOLUME
Multiply fluid oz. by 28.41 to get millilitres, or use the following approximations for millilitres:

Cups and Spoons	Ounces	Metric Equivalents
2 tbsp.	1 fl. oz.	25 ml
4 tbsp. ¼ cup	2 fl. oz.	55 ml
6 tbsp.	3 fl. oz.	85 ml
8 tbsp. = ½ cup	4 fl. oz.	115 ml
	5 fl. oz.	140 ml
¾ cup	6 fl. oz.	170 ml
	7 fl. oz.	200 ml
1 cup	8 fl. oz.	225 ml — ½ pint (US)
	9 fl. oz.	255 ml
	10 fl. oz.	280 ml — ½ pint (UK)
1½ cups	12 fl. oz.	340 ml
2 cups	16 fl. oz.	455 ml — 1 pint (US)
	20 fl. oz.	570 ml1 — pint (UK)

Medical and
Nutrition
References

Brown, M. D., et al. 2001. 'Controlling Calories—the Simple Approach.' *Diabetes Spectrum* 14: 110–112.

Davis, R. B., et al. 2001. 'A Review of Current Weight Management: Research and Recommendations.' *Journal of the American Academy of Nurse Practitioners* 13: 15–19.

Farnsworth, E., et al. 2003. 'Effect of a High-Protein, Energy-Restricted Diet on Body Composition, Glycemic Control, and Lipid Concentrations in Overweight and Obese Hyperinsulinemic Men and Women.' *American Journal of Clinical Nutrition* 78: 31–39.

Freedman, M. R., et al. 2001. 'Popular Diets: A Scientific Review.' *Obesity Research* 1:1S–40S.

Jakicic, J. M., et al. 2001. 'American College of Sports Medicine Position Stand. Appropriate Intervention Strategies for Weight Loss and Prevention of Weight Gain for Adults.' *Medicine and Science in Sports and Exercise* 33: 2145–2156.

Jiang, H., et al. 1999. 'Dietary Sodium Intake and Subsequent

Risk of Cardiovascular Disease in Overweight Adults.' *Journal of the American Medical Association* 282: 2027–2034.

Loria, C. M., et al. 2001. 'Choose and Prepare Foods with Less Salt: Dietary Advice for All Americans.' *Journal of Nutrition* 131: 536S–551S.

Nestle, M. 2003. 'Increasing Portion Sizes in American Diets: More Calories, More Obesity.' *Journal of the American Dietetic Association* 103: 39–40.

Nielsen, S. J., et al. 2003. 'Patterns and Trends in Food Portion Sizes, 1977–1998.' *Journal of the American Medical Association* 289: 450–453.

Roberts, S. B., et al. 2002. 'The Influence of Dietary Composition on Energy Intake and Body Weight.' *Journal of the American College of Nutrition* 21: 140S–145S.

Smiciklas-Wright, H., et al. 2003. 'Foods Commonly Eaten in the United States, 1989–1991, 1994–1996: Are Portion Sizes Changing?' *Journal of the American Dietetic Association* 103: 41–47.

Westerterp-Plantega, M. S. 2003. 'The Significance of Protein in Food Intake and Body Weight Regulation.' *Current Opinion in Clinical Nutrition and Metabolic Care* 6: 635–638.

Wing, R. R., et al. 2001. 'Successful Weight Loss Maintenance.' *Annual Review of Nutrition* 21: 323–341.

Young, L. R., et al. 2003. 'Expanding Portion Sizes in the U.S. Marketplace: Implications for Nutrition Counseling.' *Journal of the American Dietetic Association* 103: 231–234.

Zemel, M. B. 2003. 'Mechanisms of Dairy Modulation of Adiposity.' *Journal of Nutrition* 133: 252S–256S.

About the Author

PHILLIP C. MCGRAW, PH.D., is the #1 *New York Times* bestselling author of *Life Strategies*, *Relationship Rescue*, *Self Matters*, and *The Ultimate Weight Solution*. He is the host of the nationally syndicated, daily one-hour series *Dr Phil*. One of the world's foremost experts in the field of human functioning, Dr McGraw is the co-founder of Courtroom Sciences, Inc., the world's leading litigation consulting firm. Dr McGraw currently lives in Los Angeles, California, with his wife and two sons.

Visit his website: www.drphil.com.

**SIMON &
SCHUSTER**

THE ULTIMATE WEIGHT
SOLUTION

The 7 Keys to Weight Loss Freedom

Dr Phil McGraw

'You have a decision to make.' With these words,
Dr Phil begins his groundbreaking weight loss
book. You know he is talking to you if you are
among the millions who have tried and failed one
fad diet after another. Dr Phil is talking about the
decision you have to make to change all that. You
know those crash diets never last, and you have
to stop lying to yourself and get real about taking
control of your weight and your life. It's your
health, it's your life, it's your decision.

ISBN 0-7432-3232-1
PRICE £10.99

**SIMON &
SCHUSTER**

THE ULTIMATE WEIGHT SOLUTION COOKBOOK

Recipes for Weight Loss Freedom

Dr Phil McGraw

'Your whole family can benefit from a new, healthier way of eating with this invaluable companion to Dr Phil's bestselling *The Ultimate Weight Solution*. This stunning colour cookbook contains over 100 recipes, including: Banana Cream Pie, Enchiladas with Barbecued Greens, Mushroom-Tomato Frittata, Beef and Broccoli Stir-Fry, Grilled Vegetable Wrap and Curried Tabbouleh.

ISBN 0-7432-6787-7
PRICE £14.99